the
WHOLE BODY
APPROACH
TO ALLERGY AND
SINUS HEALTH

Murray Grossan, M.D.

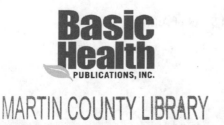

Basic
Health
PUBLICATIONS, INC.

Basic Health Publications, Inc.
885 Claycraft Road
Columbus, OH 43230
800.334.9969 • www.basichealthpub.com

Library of Congress Cataloging-in-Publication Data

Grossan, Murray.
 The whole body approach to allergy and sinus health / Murray Grossan, M.D.
  pages cm
 Includes bibliographical references and index.
 ISBN 978-1-59120-316-2
1. Allergy—Alternative treatment. 2. Sinusitis—Alternative treatment.
3. Holistic medicine. I. Title.
 RC588.A47G76   2015
 616.97—dc23
                                        2015000826

Editor: Cheryl Hirsch
Typesetting/Book design: Gary A. Rosenberg
Cover design: Mike Stromberg

Printed in the United States of America

10 9 8 7 6 5 4 3 2 1

CONTENTS

Introduction, 1

PART ONE
THE TRIO—ALLERGY, SINUS DISEASE, AND COLDS

1. The Whole Body Approach, 7

2. What Is an Allergy and Why Did I Get It? 21

3. What Works for an Allergy and Why? 40

4. Why Did I Get Sinusitis? 59

5. What to Do for Your Sinusitis, 74

6. Is It a Cold, a Sinus Infection, or an Allergy? 88

PART TWO
COMMON ALLERGY AND SINUS-RELATED COMPLAINTS

7. Is It a Sinus Headache, a Tension Headache, or a Migraine? 101

8. How to Clear Postnasal Drip and Thick Mucus, 125

9. How the Sinuses Affect Asthma and Other Lung Conditions, 135

10. How to Treat Throat and Voice Problems, 155

11. How to Stop Snoring without Surgery, 163

12. How to Recover a Loss of Smell, 175

13. How to Limit the Health Effects of Smog, Fires, and Volcano Gases, 184

14. How to Resolve Other Nasal- and Sinus-Related Conditions, 190

PART THREE

SPECIAL SITUATIONS

15. When Surgery Is an Option, 203

16. Kid Stuff, 214

Afterword, 224

Glossary, 225

Resources, 228

References, 233

Index, 242

About the Author, 252

INTRODUCTION

Janice was coming down with a cold so she rushed out (in the rain) to the pharmacy. There, she saw row after row of cold remedies: lozenges advertised to shorten colds, liquids for suppressing cough, pills for opening up nasal passages, sprays to relieve congestion, and inhalers for reducing inflammation and swelling. There were also vitamins, herbal remedies, and probiotics to take for a cold. Judy decided to get one of each and then rushed home where she sprayed her nose, swallowed the pills, and breathed in from the inhaler. She also gargled. A week later Judy's cold was worse and she was losing her voice.

Betty was coming down with a cold, too. She made a cup of green tea with some lemon and honey, got into bed, and watched a TV comedy until she fell asleep. Next morning, she made herself another cup of green tea and continued to drink more throughout the day. The following day she was fine. I call Betty's method the "Whole Body Approach."

Whatever your allergy or sinus problem, you are not just a nose. You are also the foods you eat, the sleep you get, the thoughts you have—even the clothes you wear!

Jesse was sneezing from hay fever. He stopped eating hot spicy foods. His hay fever got better. Find out why you must avoid chili when you have allergy.

Robert suffered from a sinus infection for a month. Finally his wife made him go to this fabulous masseuse for a foot massage. He felt so much better afterward and his sinus condition cleared up. Learn why.

Lots of foreign substances enter your nose. The nose is your body's first line of defense. It filters incoming pollen, dust, chemicals, smoke,

1

viruses, bacteria, and much more. Whether these substances take hold and make you sick depends on many factors, including your immunity (is it weak or strong?), your emotional state (are you happy or depressed?), your nasal cilia (are they active or sluggish?), the quality of your sleep (is it good or poor?), and your ability to visualize being well and healthy.

In this book I explain how to use your whole body to heal an allergy or a sinus condition. A major reason for taking care of your allergy is that an allergy is often the cause of a preventable chronic sinus condition called sinusitis. And chronic sinusitis can affect the entire body, including your lungs and teeth! (Prevention of allergy and sinusitis are discussed in Chapters 3 and 5.) Why would an ear, nose, and throat specialist (technically called an otolaryngologist) like myself teach a whole body approach? Here's why:

- Early treatment prevents serious outcomes. With early treatment, many serious conditions such as allergy, sinus infections, acid reflux, hypertension, obstructive sleep apnea, and bronchitis can be prevented. Imagine how Mr. Peterson felt when I told him that his cure for snoring was simply to sew a tennis ball to the back of his shirt!

- When your mind is the healer, you get additional healing benefits. If you read any carefully conducted double-blind clinical trial on medication treatments and their outcomes, you will find that, on average, a large percentage of patients on the placebo (dummy pill) get exactly the same benefit as those taking the drug. Jane's wrist was swollen and she was in pain. She entered a new drug trial. She took the drug, the wrist healed, and the pain went away. Then she found out she had taken the placebo. Frank was ill. The doctor prescribed a medication: one pill four times a day. When he saw the doctor in two weeks, the doctor was delighted that his medicine had cured Frank. It turns out that Frank had mistakenly taken the wrong medication and was taking a vitamin instead. How often have these same scenarios happened to me? I prescribe a medication. I see the patient two weeks later and am delighted that he or she is well, thanks to my medication. No, it turns out, my patient didn't get the medication—the pharmacy was closed, the insurance didn't cover it, and so on.

- Whenever a person takes charge of his or her illness, he or she does better. Whether it is cancer, sinusitis, a cold, or any other health problem, whenever you understand your illness and actively participate in its treatment using your whole body (especially your mind), you can be well again and feel good. In one study on the psychological influences on surgical outcome, it was found that irrespective of the operating surgeon, a patient's pre-surgery score on the Minnesota Multiphasic Personality Inventory could predict the outcome of a standard orthopedic procedure! When you take charge, your whole body enters into the healing process. The reverse is also true: when you give up, then your body turns off the healing process.

- Stress lowers your immunity and makes any condition worse. Being stressed releases harmful chemicals that weaken your immune system and prevent you from using your full immune power.

- Antibiotics are being overprescribed and overused. Due to the unbridled use of antibiotics, bacteria are growing increasingly more resistant to antibiotics. On September 18, 2014, the White House announced the creation of a national task force and a five-year action plan to reduce antibiotic resistance through promotion of more appropriate antibiotic use. When you learn the non-antibiotic therapies here, because you understand them and know how to use them, those non-antibiotic methods will be more effective. You and your family will be spared exposure to resistant bacteria.

Where can you get the best information for a sinus problem? Right here. When you go the pharmacy and see row after row of cold remedies, how are you to know which one you should take? If you read the small print of the cautions and side effects of these products, you would be afraid to take any of them. If you seek information from the Internet and google "Allergy," 105,740,000 items come up. If you google "Nasal Allergy," you only get 1,500,000 items. How many days would it take to look through them? No matter what illness you look up on the Internet, you get bombarded with advertisements for pills and sprays. You get information about rare herbs with strange names that are 100 percent guaranteed to make you well—and guess what? They take Visa and MasterCard. Even at the best-meaning sites for medical information, you read about the latest surgery and are advised to see your doctor. Nowhere will you find the best advice for a common cold: go to bed and drink lots of tea with lemon and honey. And, of course, don't forget the chicken soup!

I recommend that you read through the whole book because an allergy, a sinus infection, and a cold are all related. What remedy works for one often is good for all three.

No, these are not secrets of the past, revealed at last. These are not secret herbs from the island of Bora Bora that are picked in the moonlight. Every single recommendation is based on sound scientific principles that can be backed up by a dozen medical journal articles, including my own thirty-plus peer-review publications.

My goal with this book is to show you:

• Why tea with lemon and honey works.

• Why you can avoid getting a cold by smiling!

• Why you can clear your sinus problem and nasal allergy without drugs.

• Why it is important to avoid unnecessary use of antibiotics, and more.

On what page is the miracle cure, you ask? Although companies on the Internet makes millions off advertisements for miracle cures for diabetes, sciatica, tinnitus, allergy, and the like, you won't find a miracle cure touted here or testimonials by beautiful people with sparkling, white teeth.

On the other hand, if you think about the fact that breakfast in bed can cure allergy and that humming can cure sinus disease, maybe the words "miracle cure" are not so far off.

I will be describing what has worked for hundreds of my patients and how you can apply this knowledge. When you understand why therapies work, you are adding your brain-healing powers and are using the Whole Body Approach. I am confident that the Whole Body Approach will help you for any illness.

PART ONE

THE TRIO— ALLERGY, SINUS DISEASE, AND COLDS

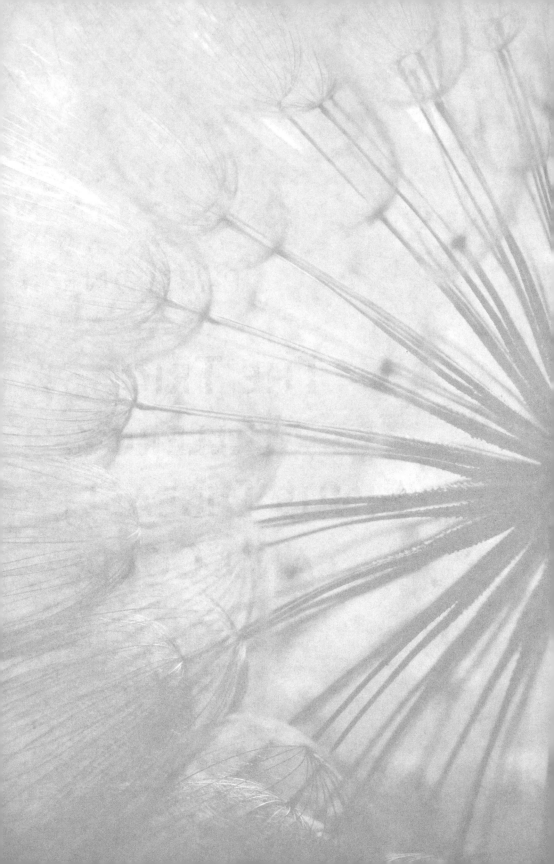

1

THE WHOLE BODY APPROACH

You are not just a nose! Whatever your nasal or sinus problem, your whole body is involved. In this book you will learn how to use your whole body for the cure.

In 1964 journalist Norman Cousins (1915–1990) was diagnosed with ankylosing spondylitis. This crippling and irreversible disease led him to write *Anatomy of an Illness,* in which he describes checking out of a hospital and taking charge of his own health, using humor to mobilize his body's own natural resources with laughter. Cousins demonstrated to us all how effective the mind can be in healing. It is because of him that today every patient's hospital room is equipped with a television and two comedy channels.

THE BODY AND BRAIN: PARTNERS IN HEALING

What is the evidence that the whole body is important in any illness? Whenever there is a double-blind clinical drug trial, half the patients get the real drug and the other half unknowingly get a sugar pill called a placebo. Typically, no matter the drug, the results are similar: 65 percent are cured by the real pill and 30 percent are cured by the placebo. The nose opened up, the sneezing stopped, and the itching eyes healed even in patients who took the placebo! In another study, even the patients who knew they were taking the placebo got the same benefit as the real pill! Did the brain do that? Yes.

Many people struggle to quit smoking. Studies with one of the newer antismoking medications showed that it was effective for long-term quitting in 44 percent of smokers. (Considering how many people fail smoking cessation, a 44 percent success rate isn't too bad.) Yet, 25 percent of the tough-to-quit smokers successfully stopped when they took the placebo. Is that significant? Yes, yes, yes. This drug with its 44 percent success rate has side effects and warnings that take up a full page. Interestingly, even the drug company noted that the pill-taking patients had finally decided to take charge of their therapy. Could that help explain something about the real pill-taking patients who didn't respond? Did they take charge? Did they follow instructions and take the pills as directed? Did they do the breathing exercises and lifestyle modifications? I believe that in any drug test, the real pill failures may not have followed directions. By not following the course of instructions, their whole body did not participate in the healing, even when they took the real pill!

TAKING CHARGE WITH THE *WHOLE* BODY

William had a painful shoulder. The doctor prescribed pills–take one tablet three times a day, apply heat twice a day, and do stretching exercises. When William returned in two weeks he said the pills worked.

David had a painful shoulder. The doctor prescribed pills–take one tablet three times a day, apply heat twice a day, and do stretching exercises. When David saw the doctor two weeks later he said the pills didn't work.

"Did you take the pills as directed?"

"Well I guess I missed a few."

"Did you do the heat applications twice a day?"

"Well, I was kinda busy."

"Did you do the stretching exercises?"

"I lost those directions."

David did *not* apply the whole body principle of healing but William did.

Researchers at New York-Presbyterian Hospital reported brain findings using magnetic resonance imaging (MRI) scans on patients who had

had stomach bypass surgery for weight loss. Patients who were success-ful and had kept their weight off for four years or more showed activity in the decision-making part of the brain when they were offered foods to be avoided. Those who had not been successful and had not kept their weight off did not show this brain activity when tempted. These findings suggest that even in weight loss, as well as in smoking cessa-tion, allergy and sinus treatment, and more, you must engage your whole body, especially your brain, for best results!

Two of the fastest-growing fields in medicine today involve discover-ies about the mind and its role in healing. One field called psychoneu-roimmunology is the study of the way the emotions, the brain, and the immune system interact. The tools of this field are relaxation, smiling, humor, biofeedback, and visualization. These are the tools you will learn to use for your own healing.

The second field is the study of neuroplasticity, or the ability of the brain to make physiological changes. Recent research shows that the brain can change in response to new information and activities and that brain cells and new pathways continue to develop throughout life. Given the right tools, the brain can actually reorganize itself to replace a dam-aged part of the brain. You will learn how to apply this ability of your brain to make new connections that improve your health.

My patient Sonia had been though the worst of Auschwitz. Those hor-rors kept her from sleeping. I explained the principles of neuroplastic-ity and how the brain can change itself. She had been receiving jokes from her family that she enjoyed. I had her spend time reading jokes, sending jokes to family and friends, and exchanging jokes on the Inter-net. Two months later she slept better and was taking less hypertension medication.

The origins of the Whole Body Approach (WBA, for short) grew out of my practice as an ear, nose, and throat (ENT) doctor, who special-izes in treating scuba divers. When you dive 100 feet under the ocean, drugs behave differently. Therefore, I must treat colds, dizziness, ear pain, and other ailments without drugs. I depend on known healing factors that will clear the ear or sinus without risking a drug effect while the diver is under water. I also treat pilots who fly planes thousands of feet in the air with hundreds of passengers. I must be careful not to prescribe a drug that will put them to sleep. The same non-drug methods I teach my pilots and scuba divers will work for you too.

WHY YOU NEED THE WHOLE BODY APPROACH

My emphasis is on a whole body approach because early therapy of any condition is best. Mr. Avery could have stopped snoring with trumpet lessons. Mrs. Baker could have prevented her chronic sinus infections if she had avoided scented lipstick that irritated her nose. The WBA is not just for sinus and allergy problems. Every health problem benefits with:

• Understanding the illness.

• Understanding what medications are for.

• Understanding what therapies and exercises do.

• Relaxation and stress reduction.

• Taking charge and engaging the whole body in the healing.

Every health problem benefits from a whole body approach.

CUTS DOWN ON ANTIBIOTIC OVERUSE

Officials from the World Health Organization, a specialized government agency of the United Nations, are now warning that antibiotics—the workhorse medications we rely on to keep bacteria and other pathogens in check—are in real danger of becoming obsolete. Daily, the U.S. Centers for Disease Control (CDC) and Prevention, the agency that sets the nation's health standards, warns about the overprescribing of antibiotics in people and animals. Antibiotics don't work against viruses but are nonetheless frequently prescribed not only for nasal and sinus infections but also for ear infections, respiratory tract infections, and other viral infections. This overuse of antibiotics not only causes unwanted side effects but also increases the resistance of the bacteria to these drugs.

Because of the abuse of antibiotics, good commonly prescribed drugs that used to work, such as penicillin and ampicillin (a penicillin-based antibiotic), have lost their effectiveness. Knowing a drug-free therapy is necessary as the number of bacteria growing resistant to antibiotics increases.

Sinus infections—usually those lasting longer than two weeks—can be caused by bacteria. I'll explain the differences between bacterial and viral sinus infections in Chapter 4. Whether your infection is viral or bacterial, with the WBA you will learn how to strengthen your immunity. When your whole body is actively helping you to get well, often you can avoid using antibiotics.

WHAT IS IMMUNITY?

You are born with a wonderful system that protects your body from harmful disease-causing organisms: it's your immune system. Although it is quite complex, what is important is that you can aid your immune system by:

- Reducing stress.

- Getting proper rest and sleep.

- Learning to smile and laugh.

- Visualizing the good immune factors (disease-fighting white blood cells and good chemicals) beating the bad guys (bacteria, viruses, and toxins).

- Drinking an adequate amount of fluids to enable these good cells to reach and dilute the invading organisms.

- Breaking the cycle of anxiety reinforcement.

REDUCES STRESS

There is nothing new in the statement that being stressed is bad for your health. Stress may be psychological in origin but it has real physical effects. Nearly every issue in the medical journals includes new evidence that illnesses are either caused by stressed behavior or are made worse by it. Stress impacts nearly all body functions. Stress produces the chemicals that impair allergy healing. Stress decreases the size of the hippocampus where memory is located. And stress contributes to an assortment of autoimmune-related illnesses, including hay fever, asthma, psoriasis, rheumatoid arthritis, multiple sclerosis, and possibly others.

Gilbert was doing fine with loratadine (Claritin). Then rumors started flying about job cuts, and he worried and was stressed; he lost sleep. He said the antihistamine didn't work.

You are designed to sleep with the owl and cricket sounds, yet awaken ready to fight if the tiger approaches. As you munch your food, you are designed to come alert and be ready to fight when you recognize the twig snapping as the tiger approaching. The problem is in correctly recognizing which is the tiger and which is the family dog. When you perceive the threat as a tiger, the limbic (nervous) system sends the stress hormones adrenaline (also called epinephrine) and cortisol coursing through your body. Non-critical factors like digestion shut down. Heart rate increases and glucose (the brain's food) leaves the brain for the muscles. Breathing accelerates. Hormones increase alertness in the brain and ready the body to face immediate danger. This reaction is called the fight-or-flight response.

Sensory input first goes to the thalamus, the area in the brain involved with perception and regulation of motor functions. From there, it passes to the amygdala, the brain's seat of emotions and, lastly, it reaches the higher brain, the thinking cortex. In other words, first the limbic system decides the twig snap is a danger, and only later does the higher brain decide it is the family dog that caused the twig to snap.

It can take a bit of convincing to teach the limbic system that a stuffy nose is not a tiger. Being stressed when there is a real threat is one thing and is okay. But reacting to every minor signal is not okay. A state of continual stress causes a buildup of stress chemicals and compromises the immune system's ability to ward off infection and illness.

Although you probably can't retire to a tropical island and lay under the palm trees to be stress free, you can reduce the stress chemicals that damage your health. With the WBA, you will learn how measured breathing sends a message to your stress center to stop the adrenaline.

You will learn how a mirror feeds back to you how to relax your muscles and send a no-stress message to your brain. You will actually reduce those stress chemicals and improve your health. When you learn to visualize with all your senses that fun day at the beach, for example, your body replicates those same good chemicals. You can be sure having those good chemicals will aid your healing.

In the authoritative psychology and psychiatry journals, there are dozens of reports of psychotherapy curing resistant arthritis, asthma, and even open sores. Did the relaxation and reduction of stress do it? Yes. In the upcoming chapters, these very important measures to reduce stress chemicals will be detailed and applied to resolving allergy, sinus, and other respiratory problems.

WHAT IS ANXIETY AND ANXIETY REINFORCEMENT?

The phone rings. "Hello? Hi, Bill! What's new?" This is the normal discourse of daily life. But what if every time the phone rings, the jaw tightens, the pulse increases, you sweat, the blood vessels constrict, and the muscles contract severely enough to cut off circulation and restrict blood flow. In your mind the phone ring may be identified as a threat–the mother-in-law, the landlord for his overdue rent, the hated boss, the threatening boyfriend. This type of response, called anxiety reinforcement, can become a harmful habit. It is one thing if it really is the threatening landlord, but suppose you get this reaction every time the phone rings or, worse still, all day long at any sound or call? Being nervous when the call is a real threat is one thing and is okay. But reacting at every minor signal is not okay. In our "jungle" today, there is no excuse to be tight all day.

Everyone tells you to relax. How many times have you heard this? Before a performance on stage or an interview or an exam, you are told, "Relax!" We have all known a really smart student who knew all the answers but flunked the test because of anxiety. Maybe you could hardly answer questions at the job interview: you came out perspiring with your heart pounding. Because of an anxiety "habit," some people build up unhealthy fight-or-flight chemicals in their bodies, which can cause serious health problems. After practicing the stress-reduction exercises in this book that type of reaction can be reduced or avoided.

At age fourteen, Amber didn't know how to drive. When her mother taught her good driving skills, she paid close attention. At age twenty-five, Amber is an excellent driver because she learned skills through practice. She always checks before changing lanes; she always maintains a safe distance behind cars on the freeway. Because these skills are ingrained in her brain-muscle system, she drives stress free, and remembers her skills even when her kids are fighting in the back seat.

IMPROVES SLEEP AND MENTAL WELL-BEING

According to a study published by the CDC, 20 percent or more of traffic accidents are caused by people who do not get an adequate night's sleep and are not alert or fully awake while driving. An even higher percentage of industrial accidents are attributed to inadequate sleep. Symptoms of drowsiness, high blood pressure, fatigue, and headache originate in sleep disorders. Poor sleep also causes weight gain; when you are tired from poor sleep, you eat for energy (usually sugars and other refined carbohydrates) and gain weight. The extra weight adds to snoring and poor sleep—a vicious circle.

You don't sleep well when your nose is plugged and your sinuses ache. Read what I teach my patients for sleep improvement. Another study (no surprise here) showed that poor sleep is associated with depression; improving sleep reduces depression.

REDUCES THE NEED FOR DRUGS
AND AVOIDS HARMFUL DRUG INTERACTIONS

My patient Jenny called me Friday afternoon about her cough. She had seen the family doctor, the internist, and the pulmonologist for a persistent cough, and since she still coughed, she wanted to see me. I scheduled her appointment for the following Tuesday. She called on Monday to cancel. Over the weekend, her grandmother came to visit and had made her chicken soup, and now her coughing had stopped. Yes, there are elements in chicken soup that are therapeutic, but Jenny's body was the cure here. Did the mind do it? Yes. You can use that principle for your own cure.

Every nurse who has worked in a hospital emergency room will tell you of a patient who came in with pain from an injury. She rushed to give the patient relief and administered the shot for pain. As she withdrew the needle, the patient said, "Thank you for that shot. The pain has stopped." Yet, the pain medicine needs twenty minutes before it can take effect! Was the brain doing this? Yes.

Every doctor tells about a patient who had an incurable condition and should have died in two months. Yet, the patient lived six months in order to live to see a son's wedding or the birth of a grandchild. The doctors didn't do it; the patient's mind directed and his or her body responded. You can use that same system for your health.

UNSEEN RISKS OF DRUGS

What about all the drug advertisements that show happy smiling people, who are taking the pill, running freely in the forest or field without problems? There's more to it:

- Any drug can have an adverse effect.

- Your drug may interact to affect other drugs you are taking.

- Any medication you avoid is a plus for you.

- New drugs are wonderful; then years later they discover the side effects.

- Deaths are reported daily due to interactions of prescribed medications.

After surgery patients are certainly entitled to pain relief. I would be a poor doctor if I sent my patient home after a tonsillectomy without pain medication. However, when patients follow a program of iced drinks, measured breathing, distraction and other aids, it is significant how many return saying that they didn't need the pills or that they used them only once.

This approach is hugely different than telling a patient post-op: "Take these pain pills–one, four times a day," period. Of course, the patient didn't feel pain, but did she continue to need more pills long after she was healed? Did she get hooked on the pain pills? Did the pills upset her stomach? Did she get addicted? Worse, did she accidentally take an overdose? It's much better to use the WBA to reduce the need for pain pills.

The more we understand about how drugs work, the more we begin to realize how they interact with other body systems. We've only discovered recently how cholesterol medications may affect the brain and osteoporosis medicines may harm the jaw. Daily, we hear of accidental deaths by people who mixed medications. You read about the celebrities who accidentally overdosed and about the mother who drove head-on into opposing traffic after taking a mixture of medications—first a sleeping pill, then a pain pill, and then another sleeping pill—because her mind was numb and she couldn't remember taking them. These scenarios happen daily.

Another good reason to reduce medicines is that too many people today are already on a lipid-lowering medication, a drug for hypertension, a drug against Alzheimer's disease, or an acid-blocking drug! Frankly, I can't be sure how any drug I give might behave when added to all these other medications. I know all drugs have side effects. I know there are black box warnings of possible dangers from certain medications. What I don't know is whether the drug I prescribe might act badly if this patient adds it to all these chemicals. So I prefer to stick to things that won't harm. Often I find that when a patient uses the WBA for one problem, the dosages for his other medications work well on lower doses! This is particularly true for high-blood pressure medications. Although I am an ENT specialist, my friends and patients have used my WBA to reduce their antihypertensive medications.

LAUGHTER TRIGGERS ENDORPHIN ACTIVATION

The reason there are comedy channels in every patient's hospital room is because comedy aids healing. A study proved that when people smile they have fewer colds. Humor produces chemicals called endorphins that aid immunity. Yes, you may feel better with a pill, but how much of that is your mind responsible for? Humor suppresses the body's anxiety chemistry and makes for better immune factors. No matter what your situation, when your facial muscles make a smile position, you send a healing message to your body. Even the act of smiling, after a tragedy, will improve your overall health.

Remember Betty who caught a cold, drank tea with lemon and honey, and then went to bed? Her cold lasted two days and she was fine! She got well because of the healing properties in the tea with lemon and honey, and by lowering her stress levels, getting good sleep, and engaging her mind's help in healing. Betty also got well fast because she watched comedies!

ENHANCES EFFECTIVENESS OF MEDICATION AND TREATMENT

Medication enhancement means that you use your whole body to make the pill or the treatment more effective. Maybe you will need only one pill instead of two? Maybe you will be cured in five days instead of ten? How do you apply medication enhancement to your regular medications?

In a 2013 study, a percentage of patients taking a placebo experienced pain relief with it. How? The placebo-positive patients knew what the pill was for; they knew how it worked; they could visualize it working and could imagine it working successfully; they were relaxed because they were getting treated. They had a memory of a previous "red pill" that stopped their pain. They got the same pain relief as the patients taking the real pill. When they took the placebo, their bodies actually produced endorphins, brain chemicals known for their feel-good effect! By electric measurement, the conductivity of pain fibers was reduced. We will apply these principles for your allergy and sinus treatments too.

Whether it is a blood pressure pill or one for infection or one for adjusting heart rhythm, every carefully conducted study concludes that a certain percentage of people get the *same* results with the placebo when they apply the WBA. For example, there is a report that for several months in England a hospital was treating its patients with penicillin and no one noticed anything different about the results. Later, the hospital personnel discovered that the penicillin was a bad batch and was no longer effective. How did those patients get well despite not receiving penicillin? The whole body did it! The patients knew that the penicillin would work; they were in a place of healing; and they were relaxed, and receiving other therapies.

With medication enhancement, the effects of medications are enhanced (as well as therapies) when you know what the pill (or therapy) does and how it works. You visualize it actually working. You become stress free to allow your whole body to participate in the healing. You anticipate and recall prior good results. You read the instructions and follow them too. It is not necessary that you understand the precise chemistry of the medication. Visualize the pill that blocks histamine (a chemical that sets off allergy symptoms) as you and your friends building a wall or the good FBI agents stopping the bad guys or even circles stopping the triangles. It is amazing how your own brain works.

In the anatomy books of seventy-five years ago, the illustrations showed a few connections from the thyroid to the ovaries and from the kidneys to the heart. In today's depictions of anatomy, all the organs, including the heart, kidneys, adrenal glands, olfactory bulb (of smell), and others show a connection to the brain in the anatomy pictures. When you practice medication enhancement, you take charge of your illness and practice and use much less medication. That means using your whole body for the cure.

VISUALIZATION: EARLY PSYCHOTHERAPY

Throughout history mankind has always had places to go to for healing. Whether it was the aborigines in Australia, the Greeks at Delphi, or the Native Americans at the hot springs, these places were regularly visited by the sick in body and spirit. And these healing places worked long before antibiotics. Most were characterized by clean air and water, nice temperature, hot springs, and plain food. Just as important was the expectation that they would be healed, boosted by the knowledge that other individuals had been cured there. People with asthma and arthritis did get better because the hot water, rest, and clean air allowed their natural steroids and immune factors to regenerate. Headaches disappeared, too, as patients got away from their problems and saw them in a new light or discussed their problems with "counselors" or priests—it was early psychotherapy.

SPEEDS RECOVERY AND STRENGTHENS IMMUNITY

Patients feel better and heal faster when they fully understand their medical problem and how to deal with it. This works irrespective of your health condition. Your body knows when you have given up on getting well! It will put out more effort when you are actively working to get well.

The scientist gave Alice the new pill. Her asthma cleared and she was able to jog again. When the scientist checked, it turned out she had taken the placebo. Why did Alice get well?

An article in the prestigious medical journal the *Lancet* reported on a study in which 84 percent of the acute sinusitis patients in one group got well with the antibiotic, while 76 percent of the patients in the placebo group got well with the placebo. Can you use this knowledge to help you stay well? Yes.

Since the placebo in the clinical trials worked when the patient's whole body made the cure, you can be sure that using the WBA with the real medicine will get you a successful outcome. No matter what your illness, as soon as you engage and take charge, your body actually changes for the better. More important, this is a learned response. The more you clear your symptoms, the better your body is able to respond to the next illness.

Tomas was a patient who regularly came into the office for earwax and allergy. He regularly used the WBA for his symptoms. When he visited me for wax removal, he bragged that now he was allergy free after using an inexpensive over-the-counter medicine instead of the expensive prescription one. He showed me the bottle. He was taking the dosage used for children instead of the dose recommended for a 190-pound adult. Here was a star example of using the WBA and medication enhancement.

Every orthopedist tells of the patient who was prescribed a specific exercise for an injured limb. A month later the patient returned and was cured of the physical problem. But, she had done the wrong exercise! Did the WBA help here?

My patient lost hearing in his one good ear. I hospitalized him and gave him an intravenous therapy. His hearing returned! I was praised as the great doctor who had cured him. Then I learned that the hospital had given him the wrong dose—one-tenth the dose I ordered. A miracle or the WBA?

Placebos work. The wrong exercise worked. You can gain back your health more successfully in every situation when you take charge with the WBA.

2

WHAT IS AN ALLERGY AND WHY DID I GET IT?

Originally, the allergic reaction evolved to expel tapeworm infestations from the body. It is thought that early people developed this defense mechanism to protect themselves from these parasites that live naturally in the human digestive tract. Although today tapeworm infection is rare in the United States, in third world countries where sanitation is poor and tapeworm infestation is common, the people's "allergy" immune system is busy fighting this infection such that there isn't much immunoglobulin E (IgE) left over for getting autoimmune illnesses like allergies and asthma.

In allergy, the body recognizes essentially harmless Bermuda grass as an invader and the IgE goes to work to defend against the grass pollen. Why did your body decide that Bermuda grass was a bad thing?

Jim gardens and cleans his garage. He doesn't have an allergy. Mike tries to clean his garage but has to stop, because he sneezes and can't catch his breath. Mike wants to play ball with his son in their garden, but after five minutes his nose runs, he coughs, and his eyes tear. Mike has an allergy. He is experiencing a type 1 immune reaction, an active defense in which IgE from the immune system triggers the process that engulfs the invaders.

George took penicillin for his infection and got well. Patrick took penicillin and his face started to swell. His wife got frightened and rushed him to the emergency room. When they got there, Patrick could hardly breathe. The doctor gave him an injection of epinephrine and Patrick recovered. Patrick is allergic to penicillin. Patrick's sudden reaction is a type 1 reaction called anaphylaxis, a life-threatening allergic response that occurs very fast and comes on suddenly. Peanuts, bee stings, shellfish, and snake venom are other common triggers of anaphylaxis. (Patrick is instructed to be sure to tell every doctor about his allergy and to make sure that this information is on his medical chart.) Patrick's wife insisted that he wear a bracelet that identifies his allergy. Also, fortunately, desensitization shots to bee stings, penicillin, and others triggers are available (more on this later).

Roberta is having an awful time with her second child, Elizabeth, age two. Little Liz is cranky all the time, doesn't sleep, and hasn't gained sufficient weight. Everyone is worried. Her pediatrician referred her to an allergist, who decided that Elizabeth has a food allergy and prescribed a very strict allergy-free diet. Now Elizabeth is thriving. This type of immune reaction is actually part of an immune system cascade. A food allergy can be seen in conjunction with other nasal or skin allergy conditions. For example, my patient Arabella had a milk allergy in infancy, developed a nasal allergy at age ten, and then developed asthma as an adult.

Your allergic reaction may be caused by something in the air you breathed like Robert, or in a medicine you took like Patrick, or a food you ate like Elizabeth. All three are overreactions to an antigen, an ordinarily harmless substance that triggers the allergic reaction.

WHAT ARE ANTIBODIES AND IMMUNOGLOBULINS?

Immunoglobulins (Ig), also known as antibodies, are proteins made by white blood cells in the immune system to fight antigens, such as bacteria, virus, and toxins. The body makes different immunoglobulins to combat different antigens. Each type of antibody has a specific defensive role:

- IgA antibodies are found in high concentrations in the mucous membranes, particularly those lining the respiratory, digestive, and urinary tracts, as well as in saliva, tears, and nasal secretions.

- IgE antibodies, which are associated mainly with type 1 allergic reactions, are the first antibodies produced when an allergen enters the body. They are found in the lungs, skin, and mucous membranes.

- IgM antibodies, which are found mostly in blood and lymph fluids, are the first phase of attack when a bacteria or virus enters the body.

- IgG antibodies compose about 75 percent of all antibodies. They are found in all body fluids and are the second phase of attack against bacterial and viral infections.

Whichever antibody is called into action, the response is the same: it recognizes a specific substance as an invader, attacks it, brings defenders to the area, and causes cells in the mucous lining to release histamine to aid in swelling and inflammation. Immunoglobulins can be measured by lab tests to tell whether someone's natural immunity is strong or weak.

ALLERGY—WHY ME?

Why do some people develop allergies? Both genes and environment play a role. Research shows that allergies cluster in families; if both your parents have allergies, you are also likely to have allergies. Overexposure to certain products can produce an allergy in some people. Hay allergy, for example, is common among farmers and those working in the storage areas. Concentrated industrial exposures to chemicals can cause allergy to develop in individuals. The incidence of allergy is increasing in well-developed countries. Correlations also show that the cleaner the house, the more antibiotics taken, the higher the incidence of allergy. One explanation, called the hygiene hypothesis, attributes the rise in allergy to the decrease in infectious disease and common household germs.

Findings from studies support the hygiene hypothesis. Children who were raised on farms and were exposed to a variety of germs and bacteria have fewer allergies than children who grow up in more sterile "sanitary" environments. In a family, the first child is more likely to have an allergy and the third is least likely. Children from large families and infants who attend day care in the first six months—both environments where exposure to bacteria and viruses is compounded—have fewer allergies.

This same theory holds when applied on a larger scale. In West Germany, before the unification with East Germany, the incidence of asthma was much higher in the West. After unification of the two countries, the rates of allergy and asthma became about the same. The people, their language, and diets were about the same. However, in West Germany, the kids got antibiotics for any sniffle and played in clean environments. Today, doctors recommend having a dog to prevent a child developing allergies later on. It's now thought this early exposure to ordinary common germs and infections has a protective effect. (One confounding argument against the hygiene hypotheses is that allergy is rampant among children in slums.)

My patient Glenda grew up in Bermuda, an only child who was homeschooled. When she went to New York for college, she went through two years of colds, coughs, and infections before she could feel well. Apparently, Glenda had to go through the cycle of building up immunities through infections. In a sense, this is similar to getting a cowpox vaccination to build immunity to smallpox—the viruses are similar.

The immune system needs to be exposed to a certain amount of sore throat and coughs to develop normally; otherwise, these systems that were built to combat infections and parasites become "oversensitive." Without these challenges to the immune system, the immune cells develop incorrectly into the allergy mode. People who have immune systems that tend to respond more intensely to allergens are said to be atopic.

THE ALLERGIC RESPONSE

Atopy is the fancy word for getting an allergy. It is a predisposition toward developing certain allergic hypersensitivity reactions. Atopy may be inherited, although contact with the allergen must occur before the hypersensitivity reaction can develop. For example, the very first time you move to an area of dogwood trees, you don't sneeze with the pollen. But next year, after that first exposure, you may have built up an allergy to the dogwood pollen. This is quite common. Thousands of allergy sufferers move from New York to Miami each year to escape the dogwood pollen. After a short time, they became allergic to the local pollen as well. These people have atopy, a predisposition to develop IgE-type allergies.

Individuals who are predisposed to allergies tend to have an excessive amount of IgE in their blood. Immunoglobulins like IgE are an important part of your immune system's defenses. IgE is the chief mediator (substance) produced during an allergic reaction. It helps neutralize the allergen. Some people are actually deficient in immunoglobulins and have to have injections of them to keep well against infection. But in atopic individuals, when IgE is produced in excessive amounts, it results in one or more of the following conditions: allergic rhinitis, allergic conjunctivitis, allergic asthma, and eczema. People with atopy also have a tendency to have food allergies.

WHAT AM I ALLERGIC TO?

Allergies are divided into seasonal and perennial. A perennial allergy refers to an allergy that occurs year-round. This type of allergy is usually caused by something that you may be continually exposed to, such as molds, dust, and pet dander. Seasonal allergy refers to an allergy that occurs only during a specific time of the year. It is typically caused when pollens are released from spring trees, summer grasses, or various fall weeds. Whether your symptoms are year-round or occur only during a specific season depends on the allergen and/or pollen to which you are allergic.

Symptoms of Allergy	
• Runny nose	• Fatigue
• Sneezing	• Blocked ears
• Coughing	• Loud sneezing
• Itchy, watery eyes	• Stuffy nose due to blockage or congestion

Less common allergy symptoms may include abdominal pain, fatigue, headaches, joint pain, and wheezing and shortness of breath with or without asthma. Allergy shows up in the blood, along with increase in the number of eosinophils, a type of white blood cells that helps tame the allergic reaction.

Plant Pollens

Allergic rhinitis is the most common form of allergy. It is also called hay fever and occurs as a result of an allergy to various airborne pollens. Allergic rhinitis affects 20 percent of the U.S. population. It is rarely seen before the age of two. In childhood, it is more prevalent in males; by the age of twenty, it occurs equally among men and women. As your nose is the organ that's responsible for trapping substances (like pollen, dust, mold, etc.) and germs (bacteria and viruses), it's not surprising that allergies affect the nose. An allergen that gets lodged in the mucous membranes of the nose can irritate the lining and cause inflammation. The nose responds to an allergen via the IgE response. It attempts to block and inactivate the offender by mechanisms involving increased circulation, liquid dilution, and sneezing. Thus, symptoms include rhinorrhea (a runny nose), postnasal drip, fatigue, and facial pressure and pain due to severe congestion. If you have allergic rhinitis, you use lots of Kleenex.

The nose is the body's air filter. It filters out all unwanted substances. The nasal passages (as well as the entire respiratory system) are covered with tiny oars called cilia. Think of these as controlled whips. These cilia lean back and then snap forward in a wave-like motion. These cilia are in a liquid medium called mucus. When pollen, bacteria, or other airborne substance lands in the nose, it gets entangled in the mucus blanket. Then, the cilia whip so that the mucus with the unwanted substance is propelled out of the nose. Some of the mucous-laden substance goes toward the back of the nose and then down the throat to the stomach where the acid takes it out. When the cilia fail to do their job of moving the substance out of the nose or bronchial air passages, then allergic rhinitis, sinusitis, and asthma can develop. It's by moving the pollen, bacteria, or any other unwanted substance out of the nose that you get allergy relief. At the very onset of an allergy, the nasal cilia actually speed up and excess mucus is produced so that you get a drippy nose.

Although hay fever can be caused by hay (a grass), there are an overwhelming number of other plants (trees, grasses, and weeds) that spread pollen through the air. Most pollen is microscopic and you are not aware of it at all, except that you see the ground covered in yellow "dust" around trees. When the wind blows, there is much more pollen in the air. After a rain, there is less pollen in the air, but then the humidity bothers you. Which you react to is highly individual and varies from region to region. Here, however, are the worst offenders:

- Trees: Ash, beech, cedar, cottonwood, elder, elm, hickory, maple, and oak in spring.

- Grasses: Bermuda, Kentucky bluegrass, Johnson, orchard, rye, sweet vernal, and timothy in summer.

- Weeds: Ragweed is the worst; others include cocklebur, lamb's quarters, plantain, pigweed, tumbleweed, Russian thistle, and sagebrush in fall.

Sometimes I see a patient whose symptoms are limited to a single pollen. But, recently, this is becoming rare. With the significant changes in weather patterns creating consistently warmer and wetter winters and earlier springs, all the trees may bloom at once. When the pollen count drops, there is still smog, smoke, diesel fumes, dust mites, and other irritants to cause your symptoms to persist. Most people, for example, who have seasonal allergy, are affected by bedroom dust from dust mites. To understand how allergens are additive, see "Allergy Is Arithmetic" (page 31).

Unfortunately, when allergy season is severe, the cilia become exhausted and slow down. This allows bacteria to remain in place and multiply, and can lead to sinusitis.

AN IRRITANT VS. AN ALLERGEN

There are hundreds of items that may irritate you, clog your nose, and irritate your eyes. For example, soap powder or a strong smell. You find many other people get the same irritation. But, in an allergy, just a tiny bit of dust–actually an invisible speck–can cause you to sneeze for hours. You have built up special IgE antibodies that attack that minute dust speck. The IgE attack causes mast cells in the mucous lining to release histamine. In an allergy, there is too much IgE attacking a tiny speck.

When the doctor draws your blood to test for an allergy, the laboratory identifies that certain IgE forms from your blood attack dogwood, timothy grass, and rye. These tests are quite accurate so that the skin tests may not be needed. From these test results, a serum can be constructed for desensitizing you to these pollens.

DUST

If you have an allergy to dust, your immune system overreacts when you breathe in dust particles. House dust is composed of small particles of plant and animal material. While this mix is not appealing to us, microscopic creatures called house-dust mites thrive in it. They especially like dead skin, which lies on bed sheets or in bedding like pillows, mattresses, and box springs, but also in carpets and upholstery. They also float in the air anytime you do a common household chore like vacuuming, sweeping, or dusting. The droppings of these mites are the most common trigger of perennial allergy and asthma symptoms.

Dust mites are resilient creatures that like to live and reproduce in warm, humid places (at or above 70°F in humidity that's above 50 percent). They are typically not found in dry climates. Dust mites don't bite or carry disease. They are harmful only to people who are allergic to them. It is estimated that there are as many as 19,000 dust mites in one gram of dust, so they're easily inhaled. Dust-mite allergic people who inhale these particles have perennial allergy. In Chapter 3, I'll discuss ways to reduce your exposure to dust and dust mites.

If you know you are allergic to something outside the home, why bother dust proofing the home? Because allergy factors are additive. You could have no symptoms if you are exposed to one thing you are allergic to, but if you are exposed to many factors, even those you are less sensitive to, together these will add up to give you symptoms. Remember, allergy is arithmetic.

MOLD

If you have an allergy to mold, your immune system overreacts when you breathe in mold spores. Molds are fungi. They are a natural part of the environment and are present almost anywhere. Outdoors, molds play a part in nature by breaking down dead organic matter, such as fallen leaves and dead trees, but indoors, where they are frequently found in bathrooms, kitchens, attics, and the like, mold growth should be avoided. Molds reproduce by means of tiny spores; the spores are invisible to the naked eye and float through outdoor and indoor air. Mold may begin growing indoors when mold spores land on surfaces that are wet or damp. There are many types of mold, but none of them will grow without water or moisture.

Molds produce allergens, irritants, and in some cases, potentially toxic substances called mycotoxins. Allergic responses include hay fever-type symptoms, such as sneezing, runny nose, red eyes, and skin rash (dermatitis). Allergic reactions to mold are common. They can be immediate (occurring within minutes) or delayed (occurring hours afterward).

Molds can also cause asthma attacks in asthmatics who are allergic to mold. In addition, mold exposure can irritate the eyes, skin, nose, throat, and lungs of both mold-allergic and non-allergic people. For many people, mold is an allergy trigger that brings on sneezing and other irritating symptoms.

Although there are 100,000 types of mold only a few are toxic and produce mycotoxins that can cause rashes, seizures, respiratory problems, unusual bleeding, and severe fatigue in people. These are not allergic reactions but rather are due to the toxins. One form of toxic mold is *Stachybotrys chartarum* (stack-ee-*bot*-ris), a greenish-black mold that occurs where there is moisture from water damage, excessive humidity, water leaks, condensation, water infiltration, or flooding. This mold requires very wet or high humidity conditions for days or weeks in order to grow. *S. chartarum* grows only on wood, paper, and cotton products and can be found in 2 to 5 percent of American homes.

Since most molds are not toxic, you should not panic if you see it in your house. Your allergist also should be able to tell if your home needs to be inspected. Certain homes and buildings are prone to making the people in them sick. In such structures, a concentration of dust, mold, or an irritating chemical may linger due to poor air circulation. The air ducts, for example, may generate dust or a leaky roof may wet the walls causing mold to grow. If the building doesn't have lots of open windows to let in fresh air (and most office buildings these days don't even have windows that can be opened), the concentration of dust, mold, or chemicals can be high enough to cause symptoms in its occupants. Various chemicals such as paint solvents, formaldehyde, or caustic powders can all cause problems in sealed buildings. There have been instances where entire buildings had to be torn down because the people in them became sick. This happened in New Orleans to homes and buildings after Hurricane Katrina in 2005.

If you believe you are in a "sick" home or building, the best course of action is to get some engineers in to correct the problem. Allergies to molds can develop into a type of sinusitis called fungal sinusitis.

ALLERGY IS ARITHMETIC

If the bedroom humidity is above 50 percent, your dust symptoms get worse. Why? Answer: High humidity breeds dust mites.

If you are allergic to a tree that blooms from April to June, why is it that when you walk in the pollen area during pollen season without your dog or cat, you have fewer symptoms? Answer: The dog and cat add to and prolong your symptoms.

Allergy is like arithmetic. In a sense, you need to add to 10 to get symptoms. For example, assign the following numbers to each allergen: pollen (4), diesel fumes (3), smog (2), and cat (2). The count adds up to 11 and you get symptoms. But on a smog-free day when you are not on the freeway breathing diesel exhaust: your count is pollen (4) and cat (2), which equals 6 and no symptoms. For most people, the equation is as follows: pollen (5), bedroom dust (4), and getting chilled (3), which add up to 12.

The reason for the arithmetic: on high pollen days, pollen can be assigned a 9; on low pollen days it can be a 2. When pollen is a 2, you can use scented lipstick, but when it is a 9, you can't. This is also why if you avoid getting chilled by air conditioning or iced drinks, you may avoid symptoms.

Factors such as pet sensitivity, dust, and aromatic chemicals in room fresheners, perfumes, and scented cleaning products can add to the severity of symptoms, as well as to the allergy equation. So too can a changing pollen count. When the pollen calendar reports that the tree pollen is moderate, the number changes to 6. When the calendar reports a very high pollen count, then that number is 10, and avoiding dust and using unscented lipstick, and other aids won't prevent allergy symptoms.

Dilbert stopped dating Georgette because he developed allergy symptoms whenever they were together. When he realized it was her perfume and she quit using it, Dilbert continued dating her. They married and lived happily ever after.

Dagmar was not responding to allergy desensitization shots. She commented that she still had problems with the leaking roof. I asked about mold and she said there wasn't any. I insisted that there must be mold and that because of her nasal congestion she might be unaware of it. When the inspector came, he found a huge amount of mold. When the mold cleared, so did her nasal symptoms.

People tend to be hypersensitive to more than one allergen. This is the reason why the allergist treats other sensitivities besides the seasonal one such as ragweed (a fall pollen). This is also why you need a dust-free environment even when you are only allergic to ragweed, according to your skin tests (more on testing later). Because dust adds a 4 to the allergy arithmetic, even if you are only allergic to a specific tree in April, you still need to dust-proof the bedroom and get desensitized to the offending tree and dust.

Cat allergy is significant. George was allergic to cats. When he inspected a home he planned to purchase, there was a cat in the house. After the purchase, he had the rugs replaced and the entire house cleaned by a professional staff. When he moved in, he still had severe cat allergy symptoms–the cleaners had missed a small amount of cat dander.

After five years, Dr. Jones finally cleared his patient of her allergy. It so happens that it was when her cat ran away.

My patient Mrs. Greenberg insisted that there was a cat at Belinda's school that was causing Belinda to have asthma attacks. The school repeatedly insisted that there was no cat; but whenever Belinda attended music class, she needed her inhaler. Finally, it was discovered that Belinda was sitting next to Miranda, who hugged and played with her cat before going to school each morning. She carried the cat dander on her clothes. Cat sensitivity can occur with the tiniest amount of exposure.

CERTAIN FOODS

Atopic individuals tend to have food allergies. These foods upset the stomach. Often the abdominal pain is accompanied by skin itching. Sometimes, in a child, a food allergy may trigger poor school performance, fatigue, and crankiness. Sometimes someone will have throat dryness and itching. As reported frequently in the press, reactions to peanuts can be fatal. Specific allergy tests help identify the foods you are allergic to. Blood tests may show IgE-specific allergy to suspected foods. For peanut and shellfish allergy, an epinephrine emergency kit is necessary. In children, the common food sensitivities are milk, eggs, and wheat.

People who are sensitive to wheat or who have celiac disease (a serious immune reaction) should avoid gluten-containing foods. Gluten is a protein in a number of grains—most notably in wheat and less so in barley, bulgur, barley, and rye. And it is abundant in processed foods, including ice cream. When someone with celiac disease eats products with gluten, it causes an allergic reaction such that the body actually attacks the healthy intestinal tract, mistaking it for a foreign invader. There is abdominal pain, bloating, chronic diarrhea, and foggy thinking. In people with non-celiac gluten sensitivity, the primary symptom is abdominal pain. Current studies suggest an association between gluten sensitivity and autism and even Alzheimer's disease, but these associations are not yet proven. In celiac disease, you must avoid gluten 100 percent. Fortunately, with gluten sensitivity, you may get along by simply reducing your gluten-food intake.

Milk allergy in childhood may be a precursor to generalized atopy in the future. For this reason, pediatricians are careful about timing the introductions of specific foods in babies and infants to avoid the body's reaction that these are invaders and require an allergic response.

MEDICATIONS

The immune system may also produce an allergic reaction to a drug. Twin A takes penicillin for an ear infection and gets well. Her twin sister, B, takes penicillin and gets a rash, swelling of her face, and upset stomach; there is concern that she may have swelling of her vocal cords. Why is there a difference? Somehow the immune system in twin B has decided that the penicillin molecule is an invader that must be attacked. After she took her first dose of penicillin tablets, she developed antibodies to the antibiotic and now penicillin is attacked by these antibodies with histamine release.

Unfortunately, any medication can cause an allergy reaction. Doctors are careful to get a history of previous allergic reactions and to avoid medications that are similar in structure.

SINUSITIS: A COMMON COMPLICATION AT THE END OF THE ALLERGY SEASON

Sandra used to get a bad sinus infection every year after the ragweed allergy season. Finally, she used pulse-wave nasal irrigation as soon as her allergy symptoms began. The irrigator's pulsing action restored her tired cilia, helped to move bacteria from her nose and sinuses, and washed out her nasal IgE. Washing out the IgE reduces the products that react with the allergen to cause symptoms. And because she didn't have exhausted cilia from the allergy, she no longer got the sinus infection.

As noted earlier, a common cause of sinusitis occurs when the cilia slow down following an allergy season. If the sinus cavities get clogged, then the bacteria-laden mucus may remain long enough to reproduce and produce the toxins that cause sinus disease. After days of allergic sneezing and congestion, a sinus infection may start because the cilia are exhausted and are no longer able to move the bacteria out. Most allergists recommend desensitization shots in order to prevent chronic sinusitis developing from an allergy. Before pulse-wave irrigation was available, that was a standard reason for desensitization. You'll learn more about pulse-wave irrigation in Chapter 3.

DIAGNOSING YOUR ALLERGY

By understanding how an allergy develops, what makes it worse, and with the help of pollen calendar, often you can diagnose what triggers your allergy. Keeping a "sneezing diary" in which you note what might have triggered the sneeze is also helpful. Most people with allergies can identify several things that they know will help trigger a reaction. But if you don't, a couple of simple self-tests can help you begin to identify what you are allergic to. Finding these triggers is the first step in helping rid yourself of allergies.

SEASONAL ALLERGIES

For a seasonal allergy, the best way to diagnose your allergy is to check a pollen calendar (see opposite). If you are in a high allergy area such as Knoxville, Tennessee, you will get the pollen count hourly. Keep a record of your symptoms as they occur in step with the pollen count. This way if your symptoms follow a specific plant or weed, you can automatically make a diagnosis. For example, when the elm pollen count is highest, you may have worse symptoms than when sagebrush is highest. Then, look to see if there is an elm tree in your backyard. By making this diagnosis, you can help your doctor's treatment. This information can also help instruct you on where not to vacation next year or on the need to further pollen-proof your house or change where you live. For example, moving to a higher elevation gets you out of the high pollen areas, which tend to occur at lower elevations. Note too that if you live on Elm Street, and you start sneezing in early spring, you may want to move to an area that is not famous for their dozens of elm trees. Sailing on the ocean and living close to the ocean are pollen-free areas.

Doreen couldn't tell one tree from another. When she was about to purchase a home in a tree-lined suburb, her sister pointed out that beech, cedar, and elm trees surrounded the house, and reminded her that she had allergies.

If you need the help of an expert to identify the pollen to which you are allergic, then schedule an appointment with an allergist. By doing a physical examination and taking your medical history, the doctor will get a lead based on when your symptoms are worse and what is blooming at that time. He or she may draw blood and send it to a lab where they measure IgE levels against various pollens, or the allergist may conduct skin tests where you are injected with small doses of the antigen. By increasing the dosage of the same pollen antigen, the allergist can determine the severity of your allergy. There can be a marked difference between a positive skin test at 1:100,000 dilution versus one at 1:10,000. With the 1:100,000 dilution, there may be a mild red bump; with the 1:10,000, there may be a severe reaction requiring treatment! Based on that severity, the allergist can prepare a series of injections or sublingual (under the tongue) drops that, given over time, will raise your immunity and reduce your symptoms. This usually means less or no medication.

Note: If you are going for allergy tests, you should stop pulse-wave irrigation forty-eight hours before the test because the irrigation washes out nasal IgE.

THE POLLEN CALENDAR

Where you live determines when pollen allergy occurs. In every major city, information is provided as to which pollen is unusually high this month. If you suspect seasonal allergy, before you see your doctor, check the pollen calendar in your local newspaper or at www.pollen.com.

Pollen count figures are determined by the number of spores collected over a twenty-four period from allergy-causing trees, grasses, and weeds. These are reported:

- Very High
- High
- Moderate
- Low
- Absent

This information is very valuable. It is best to stay indoors on very high pollen days for ragweed, and it is okay to picnic when the pollen count is low.

Alicia started sneezing one day. She checked the pollen calendar and found out that dogwood trees were blooming. She also recalled that the tree outside her bedroom window was a dogwood. She closed her window and her symptoms stopped.

PERENNIAL ALLERGIES

What if your allergy is present all year-round? Usually, the cause is an allergy to dust or animal dander. What is difficult to know is whether your year-round nasal congestion is an allergy or sinusitis or nasal polyps (growths) or a deviated septum (misaligned nasal cavity). The allergic nose shows membranes that are pale and boggy. The infected nasal membranes are red with colored discharge. However, the typical patient I see has dust, cat, and pollen allergy combined. In year-round allergy, it is best to test for dusts, pets, and molds. This can be done by a blood test that measures IgE for various products.

FOOD ALLERGIES

Food allergies are more difficult to diagnose. Keeping a food diary helps. If you suspect a specific food may be the culprit triggering your allergic reaction, avoid it and similar ones for two weeks. If symptoms of itching, bloating, indigestion, and others abate, then reintroduce the suspected food for a week. If symptoms return strongly, then you have a diagnosis. For example, if you suspect a milk allergy, you have to avoid drinking milk and eating all milk-related products (yogurt, cheese, ice cream, etc.) during the test.

If a food is identified as causing symptoms, say, avocado for example, eliminate the food from your diet for two to three months, at which point in most people it can be safely reintroduced on a restricted schedule in which it is not eaten more than once every five days. Most people tolerate a reintroduced food at this level once the desensitization period has been reached. While resolving a food allergy may not eliminate all your allergy problems, it can help you feel a whole lot better.

Note: Gluten sensitivity is quite complicated and should be handled by an allergist or nutritionist. For a list of gluten-free foods, go to www.gluten.org. For additional information, see the Resources section.

MACHO MAN (OR WOMAN)

In the movies the he-man defies pain; he runs into the burning house and rescues the child. However, there are times not to be macho. You know the attic or garage is dusty but needs to be cleaned. Use a mask so you don't get allergy symptoms (or hire the kid next door, which is cheaper than the doctor bills).

You know they say to wear a mask when spray painting. Don't be macho—wear the mask. I see too many patients who were never allergic before, but ever since they cleaned the dusty attic or garage, they have had asthma. This is avoidable.

WHAT IS NOT AN ALLERGY

There are a number of medical conditions that can cause a constant runny nose, sneezing, nasal stuffiness, and other allergy-like symptoms. Sneezing all day may not be an allergy. It may be due to the fresh paint in the office or to a new scented lipstick or to the new common cold you caught. When you sneeze every time you use the soap powder, that isn't an allergy; it's the tickle from the soap particles that feel like sandpaper in your nose. And neither is it an allergy when the brand new rug in the office gives off odors, causing you and the rest of the workers to have days of runny noses until someone opens the windows and runs a fan on the rug to clear the aromatic chemicals. Following are some conditions that often masquerade as an allergy.

VASOMOTOR RHINITIS

Vasomotor rhinitis is a condition caused by overactive nerves to the nose. Recently, the name was changed to non-allergic rhinitis. A person with non-allergic rhinitis complains of a constantly stuffy nose yet gets no relief from sprays or pills. Allergy blood tests do not show any positive results, nor do skin tests.

The nose is controlled by nerve impulses from the autonomic nervous system, which controls blood flow and circulation. In non-allergic rhinitis, a stimulus such as a strong odor causes the blood vessels to engorge, thereby swelling the nasal tissues. The common therapy is to use an anticholinergic spray such as ipratropium bromide (Atrovent, for example) to reduce the blood flow into the nasal tissue. However, patients may also get relief from azelastine (Astelin), an antihistamine used to treat allergic rhinitis, but only rarely from cortisone-type nasal sprays. The triggers of non-allergic rhinitis vary significantly and it may be difficult to identify them at all. In some people, it may be necessary to actually cut the nerve that triggers this constant nasal congestion.

RHINITIS MEDICAMENTOSA

You read the label instructions not to use oxymetazoline (Afrin), an over-the-counter nasal decongestant for more than four days, but you got so much relief, you kept using it. Originally, you used it only at night, but now you are using it almost every four hours. If you stop, your nose plugs up, you feel a pressure, and you can't sleep—that's rhinitis medicamentosa, or RM, and it's caused by the medicine. Afrin and similar nasal sprays shrink the nose nicely and open the airway. But when the medicine wears off, the nose may rebound and swell even more than before; hence, the need to continue using the decongestant. RM is a chemical condition caused by the rebound of the medication and is not a condition of personality. Treatment for RM is detailed in Chapter 14. Because of the severe rebound effect, you may need more that willpower to get over this condition.

SIDE BENEFIT OF AN ALLERGY

Discovering what is triggering your allergies is the first step in helping rid yourself of them. After that, you can then work on eliminating the allergens from your environment. It is important to understand that allergy itself is not necessarily a bad thing. Allergy is part of the system for attacking bacteria, viruses, parasites, and other organisms that invade your body. That same system is used for foreign material that the body wants to get rid of. This system dilutes the bad stuff, the sneezing expels it, and the various immune bodies make it less toxic. When you learn that dust makes you sneeze, you avoid it. When certain areas have insects that sting and cause a rash or certain parts of a forest have plants that cause the skin to swell and itch, you learn to avoid that. So, in a sense, an allergy is sort of useful. In the next chapter, we'll discuss treatment options and the WBA to improving your allergy.

WHAT WORKS FOR AN ALLERGY AND WHY?

WHAT CAN HELP CONTROL YOUR ALLERGY SYMPTOMS?

- Dust-proof your bedroom.
- Avoid getting chilled.
- Don't drive with the car windows open or the top down on high-pollen count days.
- Change your clothes and shoes when you come into the house to keep pollen, molds, and dust outside.
- Keep windows closed in the bedroom at the times plants pollinate (5:00 a.m. to 5:00 p.m.).
- Purify the air in your bedroom with a high-efficiency particulate-arresting (HEPA) air filter.
- Don't get hooked on Afrin nasal spray.
- Use pulse-wave irrigation to wash pollen, dust, and IgE from the nose.
- Get a good night's sleep. Have a regular sleep hour and a fixed routine.
- Eat breakfast in bed during allergy season.

In the embryo, the entire respiratory system—nose, sinuses, trachea, bronchi, and lungs—all develop from the same layer of cells. All have cilia, mucous-making cells, and a similar immune response, and they all respond similarly to irritants and toxins. This concept of a universal field called the unified airway helps explain why disorders of the upper respiratory tract (allergies, sinusitis) and lower respiratory tracts (asthma and lung conditions) respond to similar treatments and therapies. Therefore, it is very important to recognize that any therapy affects the entire system. An antihistamine, for example, will block the release of histamine from cells in the nose, sinuses, and chest, as well as the skin. Histamine is the chemical that sets off allergic symptoms.

All the following therapies apply to the entire respiratory system. Medication enhancement affects the entire system and so does the WBA. Consider, for example, that 50 percent of people with asthma have sinusitis and are benefitted when the sinuses are cleared. Asthma occurs in 40 percent of people with allergic rhinitis. And, allergic rhinitis occurs in 80 percent of people with asthma. Among those with chronic rhinosinusitis (sinusitis), some 60 to 80 percent have allergic rhinitis. Typically, of people with extensive sinus disease, 78 percent have allergic rhinitis and 70 percent have asthma. The important point is that people with allergic rhinitis are about three times more likely to develop asthma later in life. In short, you need to treat the allergic rhinitis to prevent further complications such as asthma.

A WHOLE BODY APPROACH TO ALLERGY RELIEF

Yes, there are dozens of excellent medications and treatments for allergy symptoms available today. Why does the one that your brother uses with good relief, not work for you? Can the WBA help?

Mitchell purchased the oral antihistamine Claritin. He read how the pill blocks the allergic symptoms. He used his senses to visualize it working. He visualized an increase in his smell sense; he visualized the pill opening his nose and increasing his taste sense; and he sensed that the pill would help keep his ears (eustachian tube) from plugging up so that he could hear better too. He found some anatomy pictures of the nose somewhere, and though he couldn't tell a turbinate (shelf-like structures in the nasal passages) from a hard palate (roof of the mouth), he looked at the pictures and visualized the pill working there. Each time he took the Claritin he went through these visualizations. Did this improve the effectiveness of the Claritin? Of course.

This same visualization process occurs when Grandma makes chicken soup for Janet's cough. Janet recalled that it had helped before. She relaxed because she knew it would help. Best of all, you too can amplify the good effect of any medication and therapy. Numerous studies show that explanations of surgery done prior to the procedure with details of "what to expect" improve surgical results. Even more effective, if the patient anticipates a reward or pleasure after the procedure, there is less pain or complication following the operation. Jacelyn had few symptoms following her operation because she looked forward to the trip to Rome she would take after her surgery.

I have been providing my patients with this pre-op information for decades. I tell my children before their tonsillectomy or adenoidectomy (removal of the tonsils or adenoids) that when they return from the hospital they will have lots of ice cream; they will be allowed to watch TV in their own room; and they will get to play with the new toy when they come home. Is it a surprise that these kids didn't have much complaint of post-op pain? Instead of fearful thoughts about the coming surgery, their attention was focused on the pleasure awaiting them at home.

In visualization, it is not necessary to be scientific. If you picture handsome men putting up brick walls to block out the pollen, that is just as effective because the brain has its own special language that is unique to you.

Visualization certainly amplifies the effectiveness of pulse-wave nasal irrigation. Users visualize how the pulsing action removes stale mucus, pollen, and bacteria. They visualize the "bad stuff" coming out with the saline solution from the other nostril. Philbert relates that he pictures the biofilm (a thick shield of bacteria that develops around the bad stuff) as a shipping box and the pulsing flow of solution is pushing that box out foot by foot. Sylvia relates that she visualizes how great her sinuses felt when she used the irrigation previously. The good feeling that people get after using the irrigator is also due to the fact that the massage action on the inflamed tissues removes the chemicals that trigger the inflammation (swelling). Just as you feel great after a body massage, so do you feel better all over after the nasal tissue massage that removes inflammatory chemicals.

Using all your senses to visualize a good result is a part of medication enhancement and the WBA. Read on.

ALLERGY SHOTS

When you have an allergy, your immune system works in excess. You are supposed to sneeze around dust. That sneeze gets the dust out of your body. The excess liquid in your nose dilutes the dust. But when you sneeze because of a tiny particle of dust, well, that is not desirable. Sometimes a single exposure to a dusty attic continues all day!

Once you have identified the specific allergen, pollen, or dust that you are allergic to, taking small increments of the specific protein of that allergen in small doses will build up your resistance. Your body learns not to react so violently to the allergen. Going for desensitization shots weekly, for months is difficult. Also, reactions to the injections may be severe: a painful arm, light-headedness, and an exacerbation of the symptoms are several common side effects. Sometimes insurance doesn't cover the expenses, much less the parking. However, this type of allergy therapy has been used for a century.

ALLERGY DROPS

A non-shot approach to allergy desensitization is called sublingual immunization therapy, or SLIT. Once the cause of your allergy is identified, a preparation with the specific protein of the allergen is made and is placed into a dropper-type bottle. Daily, a particular number of drops are placed under the tongue. Over a period of time the concentration or number of drops is increased until the patient stops reacting to the offending allergen and the best level of immunity is reached. Originally, it was thought that this therapy would eliminate the painful shots. However, it has not been as universally effective as anticipated. SLIT is available in the European Union but is not widely used in the United States. To date, it is not covered by most insurance plans. The first few treatments are administered in the allergist's office in case of unexpected reactions.

ALLERGY DRUGS

Quite a few over-the-counter and prescription medications give excellent relief of allergy symptoms. People vary tremendously as to how effective they are based on their own genetic makeup. Most anti-allergy drugs fall into the following categories and are used alone and in combination.

Antihistamines block the body's response to histamine, the chemical that sets off allergic symptoms. Medicines that contain antihistamines are effective at treating allergies. When the pollen meets up with the IgE antibodies in the nose, it triggers histamine-containing cells in the nasal membranes to release histamine. Histamine is what causes the swelling, itching and dilation of the blood vessels. Antihistamines block that reaction. Popular over-the-counter pills include loratadine (Claritin), cetirizine (Zyrtec), chlorpheniramine (Chlor-Timeton), diphenhydramine (Benadryl), fexofenadine (Allegra), and levocetirizine (Xyzal). Benadryl has a sedating effect; it causes drowsiness and is added to some over-the-counter sleep and cold products. Desloratadine (Clarinex) is a prescription antihistamine that is usually taken once daily and provides all-day relief.

Antihistamine nasal sprays can give good relief. The advantage of using a spray versus a pill is that the spray works only in the nose and not in the whole body. These include azelastine (Astelin, Astepro) and olopatadine (Patanase), and are available by prescription only. Generally, antihistamine nasal sprays work faster than steroid sprays (see following), and over the long term seem to have the fewest side effects.

Oral and *nasal decongestants* reduce blood flow to the nasal membranes, thereby relieving congestion and stuffiness in the nose. They are available as pills and nasal sprays. Two of the most popular over-the-counter decongestants are pseudoephedrine (Sudafed, Afrinol, and others) and oxymetazoline (Afrin). Always avoid long-term use of Afrin and other decongestant nasal sprays as they may cause rhinitis medicamentosa (see page 198).

Steroid nasal sprays work by reducing inflammation. Prescription nasal steroids include beclomethasone (Beconase), budesonide (Rhinocort), fluticasone (Flonase), and mometasone (Nasonex). Generally, steroids take longer to give full relief and there is concern about their long-term use. They can thin the nasal lining with bleeding and there are reports of effects on the eye. Steroid sprays are preferred for nasal polyps. Steroid sprays have been used now for decades without problem for millions. A common complaint is that they run down the throat, so it is important to follow the instructions regarding head positioning when you spray the medication. A new form of spray using a powder has received favorable acceptance. One such product, Qnasl, is a beclomethasone compound that is deposited as a powder so it can't run down your throat. I don't use this when I need to get the liquid directly to the olfactory or eustachian tube areas.

Cromolyn (NasalCrom) nasal spray is available without a prescription. It is a *mast-cell stabilizer* and works by preventing mast cells, which are found in the mucous lining of the nose, eyes, lungs, and digestive tract, from releasing histamine. For best results, it is recommended that you begin using Nasalcrom two weeks before the start of the allergy season and continue to use it during the season. For many people, this over-the-counter nasal spray gives full relief without any side effects.

The prescription drug montelukast (Singulair) is called a *leukotriene inhibitor*. It works by blocking the release of chemicals called leukotrienes that, like histamine, set off many allergic symptoms. Unlike standard antihistamine pills, the response to this expensive medication is highly variable. When it works, it is great. An advantage of this medication is that there are few side effects. It is a pill that is taken orally.

I'd like to remind you that in every double-blind study of these and other similar medications, a significant number of studies showed a high percentage of good results with the placebo. Whichever medicine and method you choose, using medication enhancement will amplify the benefits. Doing this will bring your brain into the healing process. See below for how to practice it.

HOW TO PRACTICE MEDICATION ENHANCEMENT

You can make any pill (or medicine) work better by employing your whole body to help the pill work.

Understand what the pill is for.

Understand how it works.

Visualize it working using all five senses–touching, tasting, smelling, seeing, and hearing.

Visualize a good result each time you take the pill using all your senses.

Utilize all other factors of healing including sleep, fluid intake, avoidance of anti-gens and reducing stress. Understand and follow the guidelines and instructions for taking the medication.

Samuel got a prescription for his allergy. He forgot the name of the pill and took it irregularly. He didn't take water with the pill as instructed. He told the doctor the pill didn't work.

Jeffery took the same pill. He took it every twelve hours as instructed, with lots of water. He visualized the pill helping his symptoms. He avoided foods listed in the doctor's instruction sheet. He told the doctor that the pill worked well.

Note that when Jeffery takes care to follow the doctor's instructions, he is in the act of taking charge of his illness; he is using the WBA. When Jeffery visualized what the pill does, he sent a clear message to the brain and the nervous system that engages them in the healing process. When the brain *knows* that the pill opens the nose, it can send the message to the nerve that does this. Recall from Chapter 1 that the patients who kept their weight off after surgery for weight loss showed increased cognitive brain action when tempted with "bad" foods. These successful patients were using medication enhancement.

It is not necessary to understand the scientific principles of medication enhance-ment in order to do it. If you are taking an antibiotic, you can visualize the good white knights defeating the bad knights. If you are taking a histamine blocker, visualize soldiers to block the bad guys. Or use doodles–whatever suits you. This is because your brain visualizes in a way uniquely its own. For example, you took a red pill before and it worked; the pill that you are taking now is a red pill. The brain remembers that the red pill worked before and does actions that replicate the good effect you had last time. Proof of this is that in every study, when the participants took the same "red" pill, they got the same reaction as they did with the prior red ones, even though the third pill was the placebo. Or, if the third pill is black instead of red, even if the contents are the same, the black pill may not be effective!

On the other hand, if you put the identical contents of the red pill into a white capsule, the brain may not help you get well. My patient insisted that the new generic medication didn't work as well as the prior proprietary one. Another patient worried because the generic prescription was cheaper than the previous one. He thought the medicine didn't work as well!

When you visualize the pill working effectively, the funnier you can make this, the better. Your body remembers funny. In memorizing lists of nerves, doctors use funny rhymes. Wake up any doctor in the middle of the night and ask him or her to recite the first five cranial nerves and they will recite the mnemonic: "On Old Olympus Towering Top" for *O*lfactory, *O*ptic, *O*cculomotor, *T*rochlear, *T*rigenimal.

AVOIDANCE

If you can avoid the Bermuda grass pollen on days when the pollen count is high, then you won't need any medication. Therefore, the best way to treat an allergy is to try and avoid the trigger. Although this may not always be possible for those who have multiple allergies or an allergy to pollen, there are some ways to lessen your exposure to both outdoor and indoor allergens.

Outdoor allergens: In Chapter 2, I encouraged you to use a pollen calendar to see whether there was a correlation between your symptoms and the pollen count in your area. If you discovered one, then continue to use the pollen calendar. When pollen counts are high, limit outdoor activities and take the following precautions whenever practical:

- Keep windows closed between 5:00 a.m. and 5:00 p.m. when plants pollinate.

- Wear a paper mask (such as a NIOSH-rated 95 filter mask) when cutting grass, gardening, or raking leaves to keep from inhaling pollens, molds, and dust. Nose filters (self-adhering nasal dust covers) such as BreathePure are also effective for screening out these airborne allergens. Use these when working outdoors or cleaning the garage. Do not attempt to be macho man or superwoman! Excess pollen or dust during allergy season can make you seriously ill.

- Drive with the windows closed and recirculate the air. Avoid using the convertible, bicycling, or skateboarding. The faster your nose is moving, the more pollen enters your body.

- Change your clothes and shoes to avoid bringing pollen and animal dander inside the house. If possible, keep items like coats, hats, and shoes in the garage.

When you plan your vacation, always check the pollen calendar for information on the pollen count in your trip areas. You may not want to vacation in Chicago if its pollen count is higher than where you live. It is a good idea to vacation elsewhere (best are beaches) during pollen season. Or go to higher elevations.

Miles was all set to buy a vacation home in a resort city. Then he noticed the large number of allergy specialists listed in the phone book. He checked and learned that this was a "bad allergy" area. He went elsewhere.

Indoor allergens: Keeping your house clean and free of dust mites and mold—two major problems for people with allergies—will go a long way in reducing your allergy symptoms.

Since you spend the most time in the bedroom—probably at least eight hours per night, seven days per week—concentrate your cleaning and dust proofing there. Dust proof everything. Bedroom dust is the waste products of mites and the mite itself after it has died and disintegrated into dust. (Yuck.) With a new generation being born every three weeks, the bedroom area can quickly become a major health problem to allergy sufferers. Cover your box spring, mattress, pillows, and comforter in special fabrics called encasements that are designed to minimize the amount of dust mites. Bedding should be washed in water above 130°F weekly and dried in a hot dryer. If you have products you can't wash, put them in the freezer for twenty-four hours to kill the dust mites. Keep the bedroom simple without shelves or storage and don't allow your pets in the bedroom.

Throughout the house, avoid stuffed or upholstered furniture and wall-to-wall carpeting. Throw rugs are preferable if they are washed every six weeks in water at 130°F. For windows, use blinds or glass curtains but never drapes which can be dust and mite collectors too. Keep odorous products out of the house, including perfumes, moth flakes, and carpet deodorizers. Vacuum using a HEPA machine and run a HEPA air filter in the day when you are away. (Don't use an air filter that is also an ionizer. An ionizer aggravates allergy and asthma.) Humidity above 50 percent increases the dust-mite population. Record the humidity in your home and use methods to reduce that humidity when it goes above 50 percent. Most of the online allergy suppliers of allergy-related products, such as give personal advice on dust proofing (see the Resources section for some suggestions).

If you need to control indoor mold, focus your attention on those rooms where there is moisture such as the kitchen, bathroom, and basement. The American Academy of Allergy, Asthma, and Immunology recommends the following measures to rid your home (or business) of molds:

- Clean the area. Use a solution of water and dish detergent to clean the moldy area. Then wipe off the mold. Remember to wear rubber gloves and use a protective mask if your symptoms are severe.

- Remove the source. The most common cause of mold growth is having sprinklers water too close to the house so that water leaks into the basement. If mold or mildew is visible in carpeting or on wallpaper, remove them from your home. Also, if you have a leaky pipe or roof, quickly repair and seal these moisture sources.

- Dry it out. Use exhaust fans in the bathroom and wipe down the shower after use. Periodically clean the bathroom and other mold-promoting places with a product that kills mold and mildew. Throw away shower curtains at the first sight of mold.

- Lower humidity. Try to keep the humidity level in your house between 30 and 40 percent.

- Stay above ground. In general, it's not a good idea for people with mold allergies to have a bedroom or a family/work room in the basement.

- Air it out. Ventilate damp rooms, attics, and even crawl spaces under the house to keep them dry. If you use a dehumidifier, empty and clean it regularly to prevent mildew from forming. All rooms, especially basements, bathrooms and kitchens, require ventilation and consistent cleaning to control mold growth. Also, air filters may help control airborne mold spores throughout your house.

- Leaving a light on permanently in the closet or basement or under the house can be quite beneficial. Mold doesn't do well in light.

Although this all sounds like a lot of work, the pay-off is fewer allergy symptoms. You can do everything under the sun for your allergies, but if you put your face in a dusty pillow every night or breathe in mold spores all day long, you'll never get rid of your symptoms. Finally, once you remove all those carpets and get the mold under control, you will actually find yourself cleaning less often, a pleasant extra benefit!

STRESS REDUCTION

Stress will make an allergy, asthma, or a sinus condition worse. Remember, it isn't feeling stressed that impairs healing but the bad chemicals (too much adrenaline and cortisol) that feeling stressed can produce. Therefore, let's reduce those stress chemicals. The easiest way to lower the stress chemicals in your body is through measured breathing and muscle biofeedback exercises (see below).

HOW TO PRACTICE MEASURED BREATHING AND MUSCLE BIOFEEDBACK

When you are stressed, you breathe rapidly with short breaths; you tighten your muscles to prepare the body to fight or flee. The following two actions are the reverse and send a message to your stress center: no tiger is approaching. They are simple but effective.

Exercise 1: To relax your breath, simply breathe in for a count of four and breathe out for a count of six. As you exhale, think relaxation. Repeat this exercise at least ten times a day for a minute.

Exercise 2: To relax the muscles, it helps to use a mirror for feedback. Thinking about relaxing the muscles is not as effective as getting feedback from the mirror that you are doing it right. Look in the mirror, see your face relax, then your jaw relax, and then your shoulders relax. For best results, do this exercise every hour on the hour for a minute. Use measured breathing to aid the muscle relaxation.

HUMMING

When you hum, the vibration of the sound stimulates your nasal cilia to move faster. The vibration breaks up the thick mucus that may impede cilia movement. When you know why this simple technique works, you are stimulated to actually do it. In ways we still don't understand, the mind can contribute to the healing. The advantage of humming is that it can be done for long periods of time without side effects. The lower the frequency of the hum—such as "oooommmm"—the closer you are to the normal pulse (movement or beat) of healthy cilia. The louder the hum, the more effective it is in breaking up mucous bonds and moving irritants out of the nose. Try humming at both frequencies throughout the day.

PULSE-WAVE IRRIGATION

Nasal irrigation is cleaning out your nose with a fluid. When your nose is running from allergies, you've probably wished you could just flush your nasal passages clean somehow. Well, doctors have done this for many years. It used to be called a Proetz machine, and it forced a solution of salty water into the nose to clean out the nasal passages and sinuses. The trouble is, it offered only temporary, symptomatic relief. On the other hand, ancient yogis seemed to have some success with curing nasal and sinus problems by snorting saltwater rhythmically. In the late 1960s, I was experimenting with different ways of irrigating and measuring the effects on health, and I found that irrigating with a stream of water that varied rhythmically, or "pulsated," measurably improved the body's ability to fight infection and get well. It wasn't temporary relief, my colleagues and I measured improvement in the action of the nasal cilia—the body's principle disease-fighting mechanism in the nose and sinuses. This was a big breakthrough for pulse-wave irrigation, which is now used by doctors and patients around the world. Dozens of journal articles document its benefit.

One of these studies was reported in the *Journal of Allergy and Clinical Immunology*. In it, Drs. José Subiza and Maria Barjau reported that during the allergy season patients who used pulse-wave irrigation reduced their allergy and sinus symptoms. They reported that this was due to removal of IgE from the nose. According to the researchers, not only did pulse-wave irrigation lower the IgE nasal content but it also lowered the IgE content in the blood! (The less IgE there is in the blood, the fewer the allergy symptoms.) An additional benefit was that the pulse-wave irrigation helped remove nasal pollen and bacteria. In their study using pulse-wave irrigation, there were no subsequent cases of sinusitis in these seasonal allergy patients. Sinusitis, as you have now learned, is a common complication of allergy.

There are a range of irrigator devices, types of water, and saline solutions you can use. So which of each do you choose?

Irrigation devices: Using the yogic rhythmic snorting method requires practice until just the right pressure and rhythm is achieved. Neti pots, bulb irrigators, and squeeze bottles rely on pressure alone (without pulsation) and are inferior—not to mention messy. With a pulse-wave irrigation device, you control the flow of saline solution through a convenient tip, which prevents spills, as it is gently pumped into one nostril and then out the other. The irrigator's motor keeps the pressure at a correct level, and its pumping action regulates the frequency of pulsation to match the normal back-and-forth movement of cilia, which helps restore normal cilia function.

Also, in allergic rhinitis, nasal tissues swell and fluid such as lymph liquid swells the tissues. The milking action of the pulse-wave irrigator acts as a massage; its wave-like action massages out this stale lymphatic fluid to thin the swollen tissue and open the airway. This massage-like action helps bring fresh blood into the area for better healing. It is the same wave action that is used in massage to move fluid out of swollen muscles. If you visualize muscles being massaged, you can appreciate how important the rate of pulsation, the pressure, and the direction of the pulse wave are for allergy and sinus treatment. Once the nasal cilia are restored, there is no need to continue pulse-wave irrigation. (See page 54 for instructions for using pulse-wave irrigation.)

Water: The type of water (distilled, boiled, or tap) is also important. Because tap water may vary due to your location, it is best to use distilled or boiled water. Recently, in New York City, a stubborn nontuberculous mycobacterium was reported by longtime allergist Wellington Tichenor to cause sinus infection in New York. This infection is particularly difficult to treat and is a found in people who irrigate the nose with tap water. When you do nasal irrigation, it must be with saline (salt) water—never plain water.

Saline solutions: The delicate membranes of your nose and sinuses need their own precise saltiness or else the membrane doesn't work right and registers pain. However, the correct saline-solution mixture produces no discomfort, and in fact a warm saline solution cleansing your nasal passages and sinuses is quite pleasant. Many people can use plain table salt, but it contains iodine and anticaking products that can be irritating to the nasal tissue. Sea salt is evaporated seawater and, depending on its origin, may contain fish products. Many prepared saline solutions contain a host of preservatives (benzalkonium, dibasic sodium phosphate, monosodium phosphate, phenylcarbinal, polyethylene glycol, thimerosal, etc.) to prevent bacterial growth. At least once a week I see a patient with nasal complaints that are cured when a saline solution without preservatives is used. Kosher salt has no iodine and is free of these additives but can also be irritating. Adding baking soda to the salt reduces irritation. Usually one teaspoon of salt and $1/4$ teaspoon of baking soda to 500 ml of water (16 ounces) works well.

Studies have shown that Ringer's solution, which contains calcium chloride, potassium chloride, as well as salt and sodium bicarbonate (baking soda), works better for irrigation than regular salt. This formula is similar to the intravenous solutions used for hydrating patients in hospitals and is based on the work of Professor Wilbert M. Boek at University Hospital, Utrecht, in the Netherlands, who, in 1999, reported that regular saline can impair cilia movement and used this formula to improve cilia function. My formula called Breathe-ease XL is made according to Dr. Boek's formulation.

In tests, this solution activates nasal cilia much better than regular saline. Therefore, many patients state that this works better for irrigation than regular salt. The reason this solution works better than regular salt is that the additional products more closely match true body fluids. Plus, you make it fresh without preservatives. Nasal cilia work best in a "natural" environment.

Whichever saline solution you choose—a homemade or an additive- and preservative-free store-bought solution—make the minimum each time. Keep it refrigerated and for no longer than one week.

HOW TO USE THE PULSE-WAVE NASAL AND SINUS IRRIGATOR

1. Place 16 ounces (500 ml) of warm distilled or boiled water into the basin of the pulse-wave irrigator.

2. Add one packet of Breathe-ease XL or one teaspoon of kosher salt with 1/8 tea- spoon of baking soda (to prevent irritation). Mix well.

3. Attach the nasal tip. Turn on the irrigator and adjust the pressure so that the stream is almost 1 inch high (approximately the width of your thumb).

4. Turn off the irrigator and insert the tip into one nostril. Bend over the sink so that you can see the drain and turn on the device. The saline solution should go through one nasal chamber and out the other into the sink. Remember to keep you head bent low so that the fluid doesn't go into the throat and at midline so that it doesn't enter the ear.

5. Continue until you have used approximately one-half of the basin contents. Then, switch sides and run the other half of the basin contents through the opposite nostril.

6. After use, rinse the basin thoroughly and let dry.

Note: As you irrigate the nose, you may want to use the following medication enhancement:

• Know that this is for the purpose of making the nose and sinuses healthy.

• Visualize the pulse-wave motion rocking the cilia back and forth. Visualize the cilia moving back and forth in synchrony.

• Image the sticky biofilm being loosened and washed away by the waves.

- Picture liquid flowing past sinus openings and suctioning out material from the sinus cavity and filling the sinus cavity with healthy solution.

- Envisage the massage action of the pulse waves as they milk out the old stale mucus and bring in the fresh healthy fluid.

- Recall how good the nose and sinuses feel after the irrigation.

When you use pulse-wave irrigation with medication enhancement, the mind helps the healing. Feel free to make your own visualizations of bacteria flowing out the other nostril or of the saline solution's healing qualities. Each time you do the irrigation note how good the nose feels; breathe in the air and image the cilia beating fully. This is the WBA.

TEA WITH LEMON AND HONEY

After days of allergic sneezing, losing sleep, and attendant fatigue, the cilia slow down and need to be reactivated. L-theanine, an amino acid derivative that is found naturally in green and black teas, stimulates the cilia. Sufficient liquid is needed to ensure that the mucous blanket will be thin enough to allow good cilia function. Lemon helps thin the mucous blanket to allow for favorable cilia movement. And honey, which is bacteriostatic, helps inhibit the growth of bacteria. Honey will also help if your allergy symptoms include cough. Grandma always gave us honey for cough, and the pharmacy has a dozen honey-cough preparations. Turns out that there is a connection between the taste receptor and the cough center that explains why honey is effective for cough.

For best cilia movement for allergy relief, drink approximately eight 8-ounce glasses of warm tea with lemon and honey a day. The heat from the liquid helps blood flow, which increases cilia movement too. When you feel ill, drink enough tea, lemon, and honey until your urine turns light.

Note: Lemon juice is highly acidic. Dentists recommend Sensodyne ProNamel toothpaste to protect against the loss of enamel from acidic lemon if this is a concern. Or sip the tea through a glass straw if using excess lemon.

BREAKFAST IN BED

Breakfast in bed? Believe it or not, many of my patients have used this as a non-drug therapy for allergy with outstanding success. Here's how it works.

Normally, your body adjusts to temperature changes easily. But with an allergy, the hypothalamus (your body's natural thermostat) doesn't work well. When you get chilled, instead of warming you by increasing your circulation, your allergy thermostat warms you by coughing and sneezing. Coughing and sneezing does warm the body, but it can start a crescendo of symptoms. Histamines and other chemical substances are released into the bloodstream and the symptoms continue, sometimes for the whole day. However, if you avoid that first sneezing cascade, your entire day may be free of symptoms.

The best therapy for this is warm tea, lemon, and honey. The tea must be green or black tea, with or without caffeine. You can prepare a thermos or an electric pot. Additional breakfast food is fine. Now when you throw off the covers and step into the cooler room, since your body is already warmed, you avoid the morning release of histamine.

OTHER HELPFUL HINTS TO HELP CONTROL ALLERGY

- Getting chilled makes any allergy symptom worse. Be sure to carry a jacket or windbreaker for going in and out of air conditioning, and keep warm and dry. Also, avoid iced drinks.

- Cosmetics, hair spray, lipstick with perfume, and lotions with odor can all aggravate your symptoms during allergy season. Fred and Jane came to see me in desperation. Fred had an allergy as a child but had outgrown it. Now, whenever he was with Jane, his allergy symptoms were severe. Was he allergic to Jane? It turns out that Jane was using scented lipstick. When she used unscented lipstick, Fred was allergy free and happy. It's fine to use lipstick and cosmetics with scent, except during allergy season when you must use unscented lipstick.

- Spicy foods such as chili peppers and strong spices release histamine and can make an allergy worse. Avoid them during allergy season.

COMPLICATIONS OF AN ALLERGY

Allergic rhinitis simply means a runny nose. It is the most common form of allergy. Usually, the mucus is clear and slightly salty. It is accompanied by sneezing, coughing, and itching of the eyes and nose. Once your nose starts dripping, the symptoms may continue all day. Most medications reduce your symptoms. If a pill or spray gives you full relief, it is often not necessary to go further. The majority of allergic rhinitis patients know if their allergy is seasonal or year-round (perennial), yet many need to avoid additional things like dusts and spicy foods. However, pills and sprays don't cure an allergy, any more that codeine pills cure a dental cavity that needs to be filled.

The primary concern with allergic rhinitis is if it develops into asthma or sinusitis, which we'll talk about in the next chapter. Chronic sinusitis refers to inflammation of the nose and the sinuses. Here you have nasal blockage, nasal and sinus pain, fever and yellow-green discharge. Chronic sinusitis is closely allied with asthma, as the two are seen together often. For this reason, it is very important to keep good cilia movement that will rid your body of nasal or sinus bacteria that can bring on the sinusitis.

Should you apply the WBA to allergy?

Margaret was terribly allergic to roses. If she tried to tend to her flowers she could get an asthma attack. Once, by mistake, roses were delivered to her house. She opened this by mistake and ended up in the hospital. Her tests showed she had an allergy to roses. One day she walked into a hotel, and without realizing it, stood by the roses waiting for the elevator. Then she realized the roses were there and she got an asthma attack. Later when she recovered, she explained to the hotel manager about her allergy. He couldn't understand what happened since these were paper roses, very well made.

There are cases where someone severely allergic to peanuts is depressed and the peanuts don't bother him. When he is no longer depressed, then they bother him.

Whatever you are allergic to, using the WBA, medication enhancement, and taking charge will improve your condition.

4

WHY DID I GET SINUSITIS?

If you have sinusitis (a sinus infection), you are not alone. Approximately one in seven Americans has the problem. Sinusitis is an inflammation (swelling) of the nasal sinuses. Technically, the condition is called rhinosinusitis ("rhino" meaning nose) because it affects the mucous membranes lining the nose and the sinuses.

As you now know, the nose, the sinuses, and the bronchial air passages are each connected: what affects one, affects the other. In bad smog, your sinuses hurt, your nasal membranes swell, and you cough. In allergy season, with allergic rhinitis, your sinuses are edematous (fluid-filled) and swell, your breathing is heavy, and your bronchial passages may be restricted. It is common for allergic rhinitis to develop into sinusitis and then into asthma. This is because inflammation of one area of the respiratory tract will eventually affect another.

THE SINUSES

The sinuses are hollow spaces in the facial bones that are connected to the nose and throat. There are sinuses above, below, and in between your eyes. One theory is that they are located in this manner because the eyes have to be spaced a certain distance apart in order to get binocular vision and the ears have to be spaced in a certain position to get the best information about the direction and interpretation of sounds. Hollow sinuses are an aid to speech and communication. Were the hollows filled with bone, they would cause the head to be three times as heavy as it is. We would need a totally different type of neck and support muscles for such a heavy load; therefore, the head is left with four pairs of hollow spaces in the face and skull to lighten the weight. Those pairs of hollow spaces are our sinuses. In the embryo, the sinuses develop from the same layer of cells as the lungs; hence, what affects the sinuses usually affects the lungs. All the sinuses are paired, left and right.

THE PRIMARY FOUR

The largest sinuses are the *maxillary sinuses.* They are located below your eyes and above the upper teeth behind the cheekbones. This is why your teeth hurt when you have maxillary sinusitis. Because they are so large, an infection can result in more than a tablespoon of infected material.

The *ethmoid sinuses* are located between your eyes on either side of the nose. They start at the face and go all the way back to where the throat begins. They are below the skull and to the sides of the orbits (eye sockets). An infection in the ethmoids can affect the eyes because the wall to the orbit is very thin. If both eyelids are swollen shut, it may be a sign of ethmoid sinusitis. The ethmoid sinuses can be a source of nasal bleeding. Nasal polyps can develop here and grow into the nasal chamber.

The *frontal sinuses* are located above your eyes. If you think of the frontal sinus sinus as a box, then the floor of the sinus is the roof of the orbit, the front of the sinus is above your eyebrows, and the back of the sinus is the front of the skull and brain. In a serious frontal sinus infection, doctors worry about this back wall being penetrated and the infection going into the brain. Swelling of the upper eyelid may be a sign of frontal sinusitis. When these sinuses are inflamed, the eyelids are swollen and if you press on the roof of your eyeball, it will be tender.

The *sphenoid sinuses* lie in the very back of the throat. When they are inflamed, you get vague head pains. The nerves to the eye pass nearby and can be affected by the inflammation. The sphenoid sinuses are very close together and look like one, but they are actually two, right and left.

For an illustration of sinus anatomy, see the web link in the Resources section.

WHAT THE SINUSES DO

Your sinuses don't just sit on your face. They make the mucus that helps trap the particles you breathe in every day (pollen, dust, mold, bacteria, toxins, etc.) and are connected to passages in your nose and throat that drain away this mucus. The sinuses provide moisture and warmth for air as it goes through your nose into your lungs. If the air going to the lungs isn't moisturized, then the cells of the lung passages are left dry and weak. If the lungs are too dry, then the cilia can't do their job of moving dust out of the lungs. When your cilia can't move dust out, then you cough. Inhaling steam moistens the lungs and helps reduce cough.

The nasal septum is the divider between the right and left nasal chamber. It is rarely perfectly straight because of all the falls and blows we acquire. If the septum is severely deviated, it may block normal sinus drainage and surgical correction may be needed to unblock that sinus.

On the sides of the nose, there are three shelf-like structures that jut into the nasal cavities. These are called turbinates. The inferior, or lower, turbinate is the big one that usually blocks breathing because the blood vessels here are so large and can expand significantly. The swelling can be due to nerve stimulation or inflammation. Fortunately, many products shrink swollen turbinates. The main drainage of the sinuses occurs between the inferior and middle, or second, turbinates. This space, or opening, is called the middle meatus, and the maxillary and frontal sinuses drain into it.

WHAT TYPE OF SINUSITIS DO I HAVE?

Sinusitis is often preceded by a bad cold or a bout of allergic rhinitis. Both these conditions cause inflammation and congestion in the nasal passages, and lead to mucous blockages in the sinuses—a hospitable trap for viruses, bacteria, and fungi. Whenever a sinus passage is blocked, the germs trapped inside the sinus can multiply and cause sinus disease.

ACUTE SINUSITIS

Acute (short-lived) sinusitis usually results from infection brought on by a cold virus. It causes inflammation, sinus pain, nasal congestion, headache, fatigue, and low-grade fever, and you feel sick. Symptoms may resemble the flu or a bad cold, with weakness and aching. On physical examination the doctor sees red, inflamed, nasal tissue with thick green or yellow nasal discharge. This discharge is cultured in order to identify the type of bacteria causing the infection and its sensitivity to specific antibiotics.

Most cases of acute sinusitis are due to a viral infection. Numerous studies show no advantage to giving antibiotics (drugs that kill the germs causing the infection) to treat sinusitis in the acute stage. Findings from these studies repeatedly show that at the end of a week, the symptoms of patients who took the antibiotics and those who did not were essentially the same. Typically, with acute sinusitis, you get over the attack fully, but it might take a month, and then you are clear of all symptoms. If an x-ray is taken at the start of the associated blockage, fever, and pain, fluid is seen in the sinus cavities, the sinus membranes are swollen, and the sinus openings are closed. If a follow-up x-ray is taken when the symptoms have cleared, the sinuses will be free of fluid, the swollen membranes will be back to normal, and the openings no longer will be swollen and blocked. Although acute sinusitis may start out as a viral infection, there can be a secondary bacterial infection.

Cases of sinusitis that linger on longer than six weeks are signs of chronic sinusitis.

SYMPTOMS OF SINUSITIS

- Fever and chills

- Nasal congestion

- Yellow or green discharge

- Pain and pressure around the eyes, across the cheeks and the forehead

- Facial swelling

- Localized tenderness

- Headache

- Fatigue

CHRONIC SINUSITIS

The majority of sinusitis sufferers have chronic (long-lived) sinusitis. In chronic sinusitis, the symptoms are the same as those of acute sinusitis—sinus pain, congestion, headache, fatigue, etc.—but they have been present for twelve weeks or more. The infection may be the same infection that started months ago but that the patient had never fully recovered from.

My patient Gladys is a typical history of chronic sinusitis. Gladys had a sinus infection in January and got over it with antibiotics. She got another sinus infection in March; again, it responded to medication. But then the infection came back in September. Of course, Gladys was concerned. A computed tomography (CT) scan (a specialized x-ray technique) of her sinuses showed sinus disease. As is typical, there was thickening of the membranes in the maxillary sinuses (under the eyes) and in the ethmoid sinuses (between the eyes). What happened is that although her original infection responded to the antibiotic, her nasal cilia, which defend her body, had not returned to normal function. Because the nasal cilia were moving too slowly, another infection started in March. The same thing happened: the antibiotic did kill the bacteria, but the cilia of the nose didn't return and therefore bacteria remained and multiplied, and she was infected again. At Gladys's first visit to me in September, I placed her on WBA interventions to restore the cilia, including pulse-wave irrigation, humming, and lots of tea. After that, she didn't have any further infections. Once her cilia were restored, the bacteria were moved out of her nose before they could multiply.

Another factor in Gladys's persistent sinusitis is that after the first round of antibiotics, her good intestinal bacteria were depleted. (Antibiotics kill both the good and bad bacteria in your body.) This lowered her overall immunity. I explained to Gladys that she must take a probiotic supplement and/or eat yogurt (an excellent source of good bacteria) for three months after taking any antibiotic to restore her full immunity.

Even after a patient is feeling well, with no positive bacterial culture, a CT scan can still show some membrane thickening and blockage of the openings.

One major concern with chronic sinusitis is the risk of symptoms secondary to the bacterial infection such as cough, fever, fatigue, poor sleep and associated illnesses. These include increased frequency and severity of urinary tract infections and elevated blood factors that are associated with circulatory risks, such as blood clots. Asthmatics with chronic sinusitis are especially at risk. Like any source of infection, fatigue and generalized illness can come from the bacteria within the sinus cavity: the more infection, the more inflammation, and the more severe the asthma. The need for continued antibiotics is also a risk to the sinus patient. These patients may develop bacteria so resistant to antibiotics that nothing works to heal them. A large number of patients may present with associated diagnoses, such as allergy or asthma. The causes include inflammatory conditions triggered by bacteria and fungi.

FUNGAL SINUSITIS

Another type of sinusitis is called fungal sinusitis. There are an estimated 20,000 to more than 1 million different fungal species. However, only a few dozen harm humans. There are two main forms of a fungus: yeasts and molds. The yeast is a unicellular organism roughly 3 to 15 micrometers in diameter; it reproduces asexually by forming buds. The mold is a multicellular organism measuring 2 to 10 micrometers in diameter. These organisms grow by branching into structures termed hyphae. Molds form spores that leave the parent and are dispersed through the atmosphere, where they can be inhaled.

There are several types of fungal sinusitis that may have different causes. Invasive fungal sinusitis refers to a sinus that is filled with a fungus. In this condition, fungus is packed into every sinus and can be clearly seen by shining a light in the nose and by an MRI scan. This type of fungal sinusitis is rare and is primarily seen in people with compromised immune systems, such as those with human immunodeficiency virus (HIV). Fortunately, this invasive form of fungal sinusitis is becoming less frequent today thanks to improved HIV therapy. When seen, surgery and antifungal therapies are needed.

Allergic fungal sinusitis is triggered by an allergy to fungus. In this condition, a fungus is in the nose and sinuses and can be identified by a culture, yet the same fungus is seen in otherwise healthy people. A theory proposed by Mayo Clinic researchers is that allergic fungal sinusitis is caused by an immune system defense to the fungi in the nose and sinuses. It is conjectured that certain white blood cells called eosinophils produce too much of a toxic protein that tries to kill the fungi, and that this toxin is what is making the patient sick, not the fungi itself. The treatment for this type of fungal sinusitis is to eliminate the fungi and to stop the exaggerated eosinophil reaction. New York-based allergist Wellington Tichenor has had some success by desensitizing the individual to a particular fungus (see www.sinuses.com). Where systemic drugs have been given to kill a fungus, the results have been inconsistent. Thus far, the best means of removing the toxic protein from the nose and sinuses has come from patients using pulse-wave irrigation. When the antifungal antibiotic amphotericin B is added to the irrigation solution, it removes the excess protein and the fungal infection.

The third type of fungal sinusitis is one in which polyps or some other condition blocks an area of the nose, causing a fungus to grow due to a lack of drainage. Usually, the patient recovers when the blockage is removed. When a patient uses an excess of antibiotics, it upsets the balance of good and bad bacteria in the digestive tract, allowing the fungi to grow. Although a culture shows the presence of fungus, the condition does not cause disease. As a rule, no treatment is needed for the fungus. This is a reason for taking probiotics and yogurt after any antibiotic.

The incidence of significant fungal sinusitis is rare.

A WHOLE BODY APPROACH TO PREVENT SINUSITIS AFTER ALLERGY SEASON

Jill complains, "Every year after the spring pollen I get a sinus infection and I am laid up for weeks." Sinusitis following allergy season is very common. This is because after six weeks of sneezing, the nasal cilia are exhausted and can no longer pulse to move the bacteria out of the nose and sinuses. Then the bacteria remain in place, multiply, and cause disease. The following measures will help restore nasal cilia and prevent this from happening. They will also help improve symptoms in asthmatics after the allergy season. Here, too, when the nasal and chest cilia fail, asthma symptoms worsen.

DON'T BLOW YOUR NOSE TOO HARD

The best prevention for sinusitis is not to blow your nose, or, at least to do it gently. Heavy blowing is just like rubbing your eyes too hard. With heavy blowing, bacteria-laden mucus is forced from the nose into otherwise healthy sinuses and into the ear. If you must blow, do it with both sides of the nose open, and blow very gently into a tissue. Dispose of the tissue in a closed bag. Although this sounds simple, I have spent thirty minutes trying to teach this to some people!

AVOID INDUSTRIAL CHEMICALS IF YOU CAN

I had been treating Jack for two months for sinusitis and asthma. CT scans confirmed he had sinusitis. At his workplace he was exposed to fumes from a chemical with an ominous sounding name like XR-29. Finally, Jack obtained a listing of the ingredients in the formula. The product was 16 percent chromium; chromium is extremely ciliotoxic. When I measured his cilia they showed poor function. (To measure your own cilia function, see below.)

Rescue workers at the September 11 attacks in New York have a very high incidence of sinus disease. The toxic and irritant smoke and dust that they inhaled knocked out their nasal cilia defenses. Certain cancers and respiratory problems have developed in some of the workers due to damage to their cilia. Similarly, soldiers in World War I who survived the chlorine gas attacks often succumbed to pneumonia because their cilia never improved.

Generally, exposure to solvents, paint sprays, and industrial chemicals with strong pungent odors can affect the sinuses. Chlorine and chromium products are particularly harmful. If you can't avoid these chemicals, use pulse-wave irrigation to restore your cilia (instructions on page 54) and drink lots of tea.

HOW TO MEASURE NASAL CILIA

Because the speed of the nasal cilia is so important, various methods have been developed for measuring this movement.

A research method used in laboratories is to place a radioactive particle on the inferior turbinate in the nose. A special device follows the particle as it is moved along, in order to measure the speed of movement.

A medical method used in clinical settings is to take a biopsy of the turbinate and to view the specimen under a special microscope with strobe lighting. By adjusting the strobe light speed, the actual speed of cilia movement can be determined. This strobe-biopsy method is used to determine if the cilia are moving in synchrony. In certain conditions, the cilia move rapidly but not in synchrony so that foreign particles don't get moved out.

The earliest method recorded for measuring cilia movement was to place a pill-sized piece of carbon paper in the nose and then to look for it in the throat. This technique measured the time it took to actually move bacteria out of the nose.

The method that I described in 1975 and that is used today is to place a particle of saccharin in the patient's nose, and then to measure the time it takes for the patient to taste the sweet taste. The saccharin particle is placed on the turbinate approximately 0.2 inches ($^1/_2$ centimeter) inside the nose, and then is timed to see how long it takes for the patient to taste the sweet taste. I generally place two particles, with red and green dye, in each nostril, and when the patient reports tasting the saccharin, I look in the throat and see which color came through first. Then I check the throat to see when the other particle comes through. This is an easy test to do in the office. Most people taste the saccharin in five to eight minutes; nine to sixteen minutes is slow; and seventeen to thirty minutes is very slow. If the patient doesn't taste the saccharin in thirty minutes, this suggests a poor prognosis.

You can measure your own nasal cilia movement time and measure the effectiveness of your treatment. Simply place some Breathe-ease XL Nasal Moisturizing Gel in the nose and time how long it takes to taste the sweet taste on your tongue. Apply the test times used in the saccharin test above:

- Five to eight minutes is considered normal.

- Nine to sixteen minutes is considered slow.

- Seventeen minutes to thirty minutes is very slow.

- Beyond thirty minutes suggests absence of cilia movement.

REDUCE YOUR EXPOSURE TO DIESEL EXHAUST AND SMOG

It is a bad idea to be stuck behind a diesel truck or bus. Recently, the CDC announced the dangers of breathing diesel fumes and urged people to avoid them. Diesel exhaust is a complex mixture of gas compounds and soot, and exposure to it can result in headache, rhinitis, and bronchial inflammation. This is why you complain of nasal dryness after a bad traffic commute. Much of that dryness is due to the cilia being affected.

Living next to a highway has been shown to exacerbate allergy and asthma symptoms. There is a direct relationship between levels of noxious fumes and distance to the heavy traffic. This is on top of the acoustic trauma of the traffic noise!

After being exposed to diesel and highway fumes and smog, hum "oooommmm" for a couple of minutes. The vibration will get the nose and chest cilia moving. (Jump rope and jumping jacks do this too.) Increase your fluid intake, especially of warm tea with lemon and honey. Add lemon or lime to your water. If you are stuck in traffic, close the car windows and hum to the music. If your nose remains dry and irritated, use a saline spray and/or pulse-wave irrigation.

AIR OUT NEW RUGS (NEW FURNITURE, TOO)

Francine moved into her new trailer home on a very cold day. It had brand new carpeting, varnished cabinets, and treated woods. She was cold and turned on the heat. The next morning her nose was completely clogged, she couldn't stop coughing, and she felt sick. The heat in the closed trailer had released the formaldehyde and harmful volatile organic compounds in the fresh carpets into the air and had made Francine quite sick.

When Hurricane Katrina flood victims were moved into brand new trailers that had not been aerated, they turned on the heat and became ill too.

The same thing will happen with any new carpet in a closed room. Always air out the room: open the windows and run a fan.

LIMIT EXPOSURE TO HOUSEHOLD CHEMICALS

Using bleach to clean a shower can be toxic to your cilia. Rosa was using strong bleach and ammonia to clean inside a closed-door shower. She passed out and had to be hospitalized. Never mix bleach with ammonia; the fumes are extremely dangerous.

Ammonia, bleach, calcium or sodium hypochlorite, formaldehyde, perchlorethylene, and triclosan are just a few of the toxic chemicals found in air fresheners, carpet shampoos, furniture polish, laundry room products, mold and mildew cleaners, oven cleaners, toilet bowl and drain cleaners, and other common cleaning products. Look for natural alternatives. When used, try to limit exposure and have lots of fresh air. Wash your hands thoroughly after use.

KEEP WARM

When you come in from the cold, your nasal cilia are slowed. If you step right into a crowded room, your impaired cilia don't have time to resume their job of moving bacteria out of the nose, making you more susceptible to getting infection. Moreover, if everyone in the room happens to be sneezing and coughing, the bacteria that land in your nose, get caught, and multiply, and before you know it, you are sick. In an ideal world, you should drink warm tea before you rush into a crowded classroom or workplace. At least, walking around a deserted hallway while your nose warms up can help you avoid winter infections.

Exposure to the cold and rain can also affect your immunity. When you are out in the rain and cold weather, you get chilled. As long as your skin is dry, that's fine but wet clothes will chill you and lower your immunity. Change out of your wet clothes as soon as you can.

PREVENT A WINTER COLD

The common cold virus enters the body via a nasal protein called ICAM-1 (short for intercellular adhesion molecule-1). This protein is normally present in the nose and helps regular nasal function. If you remove the ICAM-1, then the cold virus has no means of entrance. For my patients who get ill every winter with a bad cold, I recommend daily use of pulse-wave irrigation to prevent those bad colds. I don't recommend nasal irrigation for general cold prevention because most people get regular colds that do not lead to sinusitis. Instead, to prevent illness during the winter cold make sure to eat yogurt and take probiotic supplements. These will strengthen your immune system.

Note: You may or may not have a fever with a common cold. If the fever is slight, I don't recommend drugs to lower it (a fever means your body is fighting the virus). It means you should stay in bed. If the fever is quite high, it's time to see a doctor.

HOW TO FIGHT INFECTION WHEN YOU FLY

Getting a cold every time you fly is a problem that keeps certain people grounded. My patient Evelyn had not flown in five years because she would be sick for a week after each flight. And as though fate was against her, she always managed to sit next to the person on the flight who was coughing and had never heard of tissues. Most airplanes recirculate the cabin air today. Still, a comparison of flights with filtered and unfiltered fresh air showed that there was little observable difference–both found about 20 percent incidence of common colds among passengers who fly. Many of these colds are preventable.

On commercial flights, the air is quite dry, which dries the nose. So, even if the cilia do their best, the mucus is still too thick to move. Because it is stagnant, bacteria and viruses can multiply and enter the body. Therefore, it is vital to take in adequate fluids during the flight–but not alcohol or coffee (which have a diurctic effect). What is needed is warm water, preferably a peppermint tea with mint–and lots of it! Lemon and honey are also good. Warm tea, with or without caffeine, helps move the cilia. Ice drinks slow the cilia. Since the key here is moisturizing the nose, saline nasal sprays (free of preservatives) and a nasal moisturizing gel are beneficial.

Many ordinary medications can dry the nose. For my patients I find that certain types of nasal moisturizing gels are best for flights. The reason the gels are best is that in order for the viruses and bacteria to enter the body, they must attach to a nasal protein called ICAM-1. A gel with the appropriate formulation can help to prevent this attachment by acting as a shield to prevent the germs from reaching the nasal membrane. The best gels have ingredients that allow the body's natural defense elements, such as lysozymes and other disease-fighting white blood cells, to travel to where they are needed to fight invading organisms. For example, Breathe-ease XL Nasal Moisturizing Gel is a water-soluble gel that can cover the nasal membranes and provide moisture to the area. Apply it before boarding and about every three to four hours during flight. (An alternative is to use saline-type sprays before boarding and about every two hours during the flight.) After a long flight, use a saline spray to stimulate nasal cilia that haven't recovered from the dry air in the flight.

SMILE

Science has shown that smiling helps your immune system work better. Smiling reduces the body's stress response. When you smile, it sends a signal to the stress center in your brain that there is no stressor. As a result, fewer stress chemicals are released into the body and immunity is increased. In the high fashion stores, salespeople are taught to smile to their customers. The sales do go up and sick days go down too!

Feeling depressed weakens the immune system. The muscle action of smiling can reduce the unwanted systemic effects of depression and improve your mood.

Yoko Ono, widow of John Lennon, tells how she made a smile on her face, despite bereavement, in order to prevent illness.

GET A GOOD NIGHT'S SLEEP

Good sleep is essential for sinus health. It helps to establish a regular sleep routine and schedule. Forget the eleven o'clock news and get to bed earlier. The more formal your routine before going to sleep, such as brushing your hair, taking a bath, moisturizing your face, and so on, and the more consistent your bedtime, the better sleep you get. The better your sleep, the better you will overcome any illness by your natural immunity.

For a good sleep, make your bedroom sleep-friendly. Keep the room at a steady warm temperature in winter. Overhead lights need to be out. If you need to go to the bathroom in the middle of the night, avoid turning on an overhead light; otherwise, your sleep center will interpret that as being daylight and you will have difficulty going back to sleep. Some people sleep better with a distraction like a water-bubbling fountain, soft music, or even a dull TV show—see which works for you.

DIAGNOSING SINUSITIS

To diagnose sinusitis requires a visit to the doctor's office. There, you'll likely be asked for a history of your symptoms:

How many colds do you get a year? Are they severe? Do they last several weeks?

How often did you receive antibiotics past year? Were the antibiotics for sinusitis?

Can you tell me more about your headaches?

What about face pain?

Any coughing or wheezing? A history of allergies?

The typical sinus history is someone who gets frequent colds that lead to lingering nasal blockage, facial pain, yellow-green discharge, coughing, and awful thick slime that runs down the throat. Fever is generally mild. Sinus headaches respond to over-the-counter pain medications whereas dental jaw pain does not.

Doctors also gather physical clues. You'll likely be asked:

Is there localized pain in the bone that is the roof of the eye socket? (That indicates tenderness at the frontal sinuses above the eye.)

Is there tenderness between the eyes? (That is often due to inflammation of the ethmoid sinuses located between the eyes.)

Is there tenderness of the cheeks? (That suggests a problem in the maxillary sinuses, below the eyes.) The teeth will be checked for disease because the nerve to the upper teeth is the same nerve as the one to the maxillary sinus.

Examine the nose. Where is the swelling? Is the swelling pale almost gray? (That is the color of allergy.) Is it red? (That is the color of inflammation.) What color is the drainage? If it is green-yellow that is caused by bacteria infection and needs to be cultured by a lab.

Doctors also look for polyps, grape-like bundles that block breathing.

With a tiny telescope called a nasal endoscope, the openings of the sinuses are visualized. If the opening of the right maxillary sinus is blocked, and patient has pain in that sinus, then the diagnosis is made: it's sinusitis.

5

WHAT TO DO FOR YOUR SINUSITIS

HOW CAN YOU HELP CLEAR A SINUS CONDITION?

- Hum louder.
- Drink lots of warm green tea with lemon and honey.
- Practice measured breathing.
- Visualize going to a healing place.
- Get adequate rest.
- Use pulse-wave irrigation.

- Add xylitol to saline solution to reduce bacteria.
- Add an antibiotic or anti-fungal to saline solution if your doctor recommends it.
- Replace the good bacteria removed by the antibiotics with yogurt and probiotics.

Sinusitis is a common diagnosis. Annually, it accounts for 20 million office visits in the United States and between 15 and 21 percent of annual antibiotic prescriptions. Approximately, sinusitis is common, affecting 37 million Americans every year, and most of these cases could be prevented by restoring the nasal cilia! Under normal conditions, the nasal cilia in your nose and chest act like tiny paddles to move bacteria out of the nose. This cilia movement keeps you healthy because the bacteria don't stay in the nose or chest long enough to multiply and produce a sinus infection or respiratory problem. A sign that they are not working is extreme dryness in the nose or green-yellow discharge.

When you have a fever, localized pain, nasal congestion, and fatigue for twelve weeks or more, that signifies chronic sinusitis.

A WHOLE BODY APPROACH
TO CLEAR YOUR SINUS CONDITION

The standard treatment of chronic sinusitis is six weeks of antibiotics, plus a nasal decongestant and often a steroid nose spray. Despite this arsenal, many people's sinus condition continues to return. But the patients I see are more like Sam.

Sam came to me because he had been on antibiotics for two six-week courses, and the doctor thought he might need a third six-week course. He brought his CT scan, which showed congestion in several sinus cavities. He showed evidence of poor cilia function, mildly inflamed nasal tissue, yellow-tinged mucus in the back of his throat, and mild "bumps" or lymph tissue in the back of his throat. Clearly, his problem was one of poor nasal cilia function. His cilia were not moving bacteria out of the nose; therefore, the bacteria remained in place and multiplied.

He was put on measures to return his cilia to normal: humming, tea with lemon and honey, and pulse-wave irrigation. The irrigation was at a pulse rate best to restore nasal cilia. The salt mix was one designed to speed cilia. He was also advised to eat yogurt and to take probiotic supplements to replace the good bacteria removed by the antibiotics.

I reexamined Sam in a week. He was improved. His culture was back from the lab with the antibiotic sensitivity test showing that it was susceptible to ciprofloxin (Cipro). I could have added the indicated antibiotic to the saline solution; however, I decided to continue without an antibiotic. After three weeks of this course, Sam's sinus condition was sufficiently cleared so that further irrigation was not necessary. Once the nasal cilia are normal, they don't need to be more normal.

As mentioned earlier, officials from the World Health Organization, are now warning that antibiotics—the workhorse medications we rely on to keep bacteria and other pathogens in check—are in real danger of becoming obsolete due to their overuse for viruses or to the common practice of taking less than the prescribed amount. Bacteria are smart:

as soon as the antibiotic starts to affect them, they start altering their chemistry to combat that "poison." When insufficient doses of the antibiotic are given, they are able to develop immunity to that drug.

What to do? You still need to take an antibiotic when you have a serious bacterial infection but . . . most infections are viral. The better your inborn resistance, the better you can clear an infection without the need of an antibiotic.

HUM

As you now know, when you hum that vibration is transmitted to your cilia and they vibrate too! Normally, nasal cilia move in a coordinated manner as they whip back and forth. If the mucus thickens that movement is impaired. The bacteria get trapped, multiply, and produce toxins that make you sick; they also produce biofilm—a protective coating that can keep an antibiotic and good white blood cell defenders from getting at them.

Humming breaks the mucus bonds that compose this thick mucus. Try different tones. Place your fingers alongside your nose to feel the vibration. Humming at a low pitch, such as "oooommmm," gets the slow cilia moving. The vibration helps synchronize their movement, which is important. A louder volume provides more energy to break up the thick mucus. Try humming the vowels: A, E, I, O, U.

DRINK LIQUIDS, LIQUIDS, AND MORE LIQUIDS

You need an adequate intake of water in order to keep your mucus thin enough for good cilia movement. Lemon and lime drinks thin your mucus. Drink lots of water with a squeeze of lemon or lime. Warm liquids are also essential because they stimulate the cilia. Aim to have several cups of green and black tea (with or without caffeine) several times a day. These teas contain the amino acid derivative L-theanine, an important factor in healing and immunity. Chicken soup has cilio-support elements too (see my favorite recipe on page 93). For a sinus infection, drink enough liquids so that your urine turns light.

Avoid iced liquids as they slow the cilia, chill you, and can aggravate your symptoms.

Note: Because the juice of lemons and limes is acidic and can dissolve tooth enamel, it's a good idea to use an enamel replacement toothpaste such as Sensodyne Pro-Enamel. If you drink lemon or lime through a straw, that saves the tooth enamel.

WHAT IMPAIRS SINUS HEALING

- Having an allergy at the same time as the sinusitis.

- Heavy nose blowing.

- Inadequate sleep.

- Factors of lowered immunity (poor sleep; exposure to mold, dust, diesel exhaust, and formaldehyde).

- Reduced cilia function.

- Anatomical factors such as blockage to drainage and breathing.

LOWER THAT STRESS

Stress reduces your immunity; therefore for any illness, it is important to reduce stress factors. Practice measured breathing: breathe in for a count of four and out for a count of six. As you exhale, let that be a signal to relax the whole body. Repeat this breathing exercise at least ten times a day for a minute. When you are under tension and stress, measured breathing can help you relax quickly. The importance of this simple exercise should not be underestimated. While doing it you are learning how to regulate your autonomic nervous system—the part of the nervous system that controls autonomic functions like breathing and heart rate previously thought to be involuntary. For additional stress reduction suggestions, see the following page.

Ten Stress Reduction Actions from *Stressed? Anxiety? Your Cure Is in the Mirror*

The following actions are best performed in sequence. At first do each action for about a minute. Later, you may choose to do one action every hour for a minute throughout the day. What is important is daily repetition in order to lay down new circuitry (that's neuroplasticity).

1. Breathe in for a count of four. The incoming air fuels your body and you feel stronger.

2. Breathe out for a count of six. The outgoing air helps relieve your body of all anxiety and you feel less stress. Some anxiety leaves in the air and some leaves through your feet into the ground.

3. Silently count your breathing with emphasis on relaxing as you exhale for a count of six.

4. Look in a mirror and see your face relax. Recall pleasant relaxing scenes.

5. Look in the mirror and see your jaw relax. Don't open your jaw. Let it open by relaxing your muscles.

6. Continue looking in the mirror. Now see your shoulders relax.

7. Recall a time and a place before your current condition when you were fully relaxed and having fun. Use all five senses. That way you replicate the good chemistry you had then.

8. Now starting with your feet, contract and relax each muscle as you move progressively up the torso. Then, repeat the action from your hands up to the shoulders.

9. Raise your index finger. Take three measured breaths–in for a count of four and out for a count of six. At the end of the third breath, drop your finger. Let that be a gong or a drum signal to fully relax your body.

10. Take a trip to an imaginary perfect place of healing in the future where they fill you with wonderful vitamins and music that relaxes you and dispels any stress.

Actions 1, 2, and 3 are stress-reduction techniques. When you are anxious, your breath speeds up. By slowing your breath, you send an unmistakable signal to your stress center that there is no stress. Counting is very important. When you count, you are not thinking about the taxes, the parking, and so on.

Actions 4, 5, and 6 are based on principles of biofeedback. When you use a mirror, the mirror feeds back to you if you are doing it right. If you are extremely rich, you can also buy a device that measures your muscle electricity and feeds back to you when you are relaxed.

Action 8 is based on the work of physician and psychiatrist Edmund Jacobson over half a century ago. His development of the muscle relaxation technique called progressive relaxation has been demonstrated consistently to manage stress and stress-related conditions like insomnia and anxiety, reduce hypertension, and improve overall well-being.

Action 9 can be used in any stress situation. For example, my scuba-diving patients use this to reduce wasted air while diving; they can remain underwater much longer.

And what is the evidence that actions 7 and 10 work? And how does visualization work? Psychologist Ellen Langer, a professor at Harvard University, had a group of seventy year olds placed in an artificial environment surrounded by mementos of twenty-five years earlier (a black-and-white television, a vintage radio, *Life* magazines, etc.). They were asked to pretend using all five senses that they were young men again. For one week, they discussed issues of that time, watched movies, and listened to radio programs, and so on. Before and after the experiment, the men took a battery of cognitive and physical tests. By every measurement their chemistry was changed to that period of men twenty-five years younger. This same action of going back before you had the illness, in you mind, using all five senses, has been replicated by other scientists with similar results. Using five senses to visualize a time of good health directs the body to replicate that good chemistry. To read more about Dr. Langer's unconventional studies, see her book *Counterclockwise* (2010).

GET A GOOD NIGHT'S SLEEP

It is hard to sleep with a plugged nose. Inhaling menthol from a Vick's vapor inhaler or a Benzedrex inhaler helps. Another simple way to help the breathing passages remain open while you sleep is to gently adhere a half-inch of medical tape to the underside of your nose, then stretch and secure the other end of the tape to the dorsum (bridge) of your between the eyes. First try elevating the tip of the nose to see if this opens the airway.

If you nose is severely blocked with heavy drainage, use one of the inhalers mentioned above to unplug it, and then do pulse-wave irrigation (discussed next). This combination usually will open the nasal passages because the pulse-wave action massages or milks out swollen tissue. It also helps remove factors like kinase, a protein that promotes inflammation. When those factors are reduced, you sleep better.

WHY IS PULSE-WAVE IRRIGATION IMPORTANT?

Where studies in which an antibiotic versus a placebo is used, there are fewer symptoms in the antibiotic-taking patients at the end of therapy; but the difference is not huge. It differs by only 10 percent. However, 80 percent of the antibiotic-takers also experienced side effects, including diarrhea, vaginal and oral thrush, and others. The researchers questioned whether the 10 percent advantage gained by using antibiotics justified the side effects? Unfortunately, the placebo (no antibiotic) patients did not have the advantage of the WBA, including restoration of cilia, removal of pus from nose and sinuses, medication enhancement, and the other remedies we have explored. The other huge advantage of avoiding the antibiotics is that you don't build up a drug-resistant organism.

USE PULSE-WAVE IRRIGATION

The most effective measure you can take to treat sinusitis is to use pulse-wave irrigation daily with a saltwater solution. Irrigating the nasal and sinus passages helps wash out some of the bacteria. The fewer the bacteria there are, the more opportunity there will be for your body's immune defenders to handle the bacterial invaders. Aim to irrigate your sinuses two times a day when you have chronic sinusitis. See page 54 for instructions on how to prepare the pulse-wave irrigator and how to use it.

As mentioned in Chapter 3, the type of irrigator you use is important. There are frequent articles in the press today about the negative effects of irrigation with the neti pot (a teapot-like device). Is it any wonder that the number one question I get asked is about constant use of the neti pot for allergic rhinitis or chronic sinusitis. Cardiothoracic surgeon and TV personality Mehmet Oz recommends irrigating with the neti pot. This device may remove some nasal mucus but, unfortunately, it won't clean out sinus contents. A serious problem with the neti pot and other devices like the bulb irrigator or the squeeze bottle is that they can create flowback—meaning that the contaminated mucus from the nose flows back into the spout. Left in place, this is a perfect place for the bacteria to multiply and to be reintroduced into the nose and sinuses. Essentially, you are washing bacteria from one part of your nose to another with bacteria from your own nose.

In a 2010 article in the *American Journal of Rhinology and Allergy,* Dr. John Lee and his colleagues reported that even after giving careful instruction to their patients, 50 percent showed infection due to *Pseudomonas aeroginosa* in the irrigating instrument. In that same year in the journal *Laryngoscope,* Dr. Mark Keen reported on his study in which he gave his patients with chronic sinusitis a fresh bottle to irrigate with at every two-week visit along with instructions for keeping it clean. Within two weeks of use, 97 percent of the bottles showed bacterial contamination and 50 percent were infected with *Staphylococcus aureus,* the type of bacteria that cause most staph infections. Four of six irrigation bottles when tested for contamination showed biofilm.

In 2012, the FDA reported on two cases in Louisiana in which patients died after contracting infections from using neti pots. In both cases, tap water was used containing an amoeba present in ponds called *Naegleria foweri.* It is conjectured that there was flowback, which made an ideal breeding spot for the organisms. The combination of concentrated organisms, and the head leaning to the side, caused a pressure build up at the roof of the nasal cavity where the openings to the organ of smell are located, so that the pressure pushed the infected material into the brain.

Dr. Talal M. Nsouli, a prominent Washington, D.C.-based allergist, found that about 60 percent of his patients had an increase in sinus infections with continued use of neti pots over several months time. When they stopped daily irrigation with the pot, he reported that his patients got well!

Besides this serious problem of flowback, neither neti pots nor squeeze bottles remove sinus contents. Normally, the frontal, maxillary, and sphenoid sinuses drain by way of small openings. In order to best remove these contents, you need a steady stream and pressure past the opening. This steady flow creates a "Bernoulli effect," a vacuum effect that sucks out the sinus contents. With a pot or squeeze bottle you don't get a steady stream at a steady pressure.

When you use a neti pot or a squeeze bottle, it is difficult to control the pressure; it can be too high or too low. Too high a pressure can be harmful by pushing nasal bacteria into healthy areas including the ear; too low a pressure doesn't remove unwanted nasal contents. In using various devices, you lay the head to the side. This puts the nasal opening to the ear, the eustachian tube, in a dependent position so that liquid accumulates at that opening and may travel to the middle ear. I regularly see patients who developed ear problems because of this.

In contrast, pulse-wave irrigation is provided in a steady flow. This steady flow past a sinus opening is effective for suctioning out the sinus contents. In addition, with pulse-wave irrigation, the pulsing action pumps saline into the sinuses and displaces the contents. A pulse-wave nasal irrigator allows you to adjust the pressure so that it is comfortable. This also makes it easy for children to use. With a pulse-wave irrigator, you bend into the sink so you see the sink drain; you hold your head to the midline. That way you avoid the liquid going into the ear like it does with the neti pot, where you are required to keep your head to the side.

After you irrigate, your sinuses will contain the saline solution. This solution has displaced the mucus and bacteria that were in your sinuses.

In about ten minutes, the cilia will move the saline out of the nose. This shows that the saline went where you wanted it to go—into the sinus cavities. Once the cilia recover normal cilia speed, then the body can defend itself. Once the cilia move normally, there is no need for more irrigation—you don't need the cilia to be more normal. This is an important difference, instead of using pots and squeeze bottles daily with risk of re-infection, you cure the condition by restoring good nasal cilia.

DAILY IRRIGATION: IRRIGATE WISELY

There are protective enzymes such lysozymes and lactoferrin in your nose that serve as your first line of defense against infections. There are antibodies in your nose to fight bacteria. There are good disease-fighting white cells, too. Daily irrigation removes a portion of bad bacteria from your nose, but it also removes these important substances as well. For example, if you irrigate at eight o'clock and get bacteria landing in your nose at ten o'clock, you are missing the defenders of the nose. So, unless you have a full-blown infection, if you don't have a reason to irrigate, don't do it! With the pulse-wave action, you stop irrigating as soon as your cilia return to normal function. With less irrigation needed, you preserve all the good enzymes and disease fighters.

PULSE-WAVE IRRIGATION WITH XYLITOL
FOR LOW-GRADE INFECTIONS

There are conditions where even pulse-wave irrigation at the "harmonius" rate of pulsation ideal for restoring cilia movement may not be sufficient, and my patients continue to have a low-grade sinus infection. They don't seem to clear up completely. They may have too few nasal cilia to effectively sweep away the bacteria and, therefore, the bacteria multiply despite the best efforts of the cilia. For example, someone who has had radiation therapy to the head may have their cilia function reduced. Or someone who has had too much nasal turbinate material removed, as in empty nose syndrome (a serious complication of sinus surgery), may be constantly battling a low-grade infection. Or a person's cilia may be impaired by excessive toxins or the mucus layer may be too thick to allow cilia to paddle away bacteria, or biofilm may be creating a gelatinous shield around the bacteria, making it impervious to the simple flush. In these types of situations, I recommend adding xylitol to the nasal irrigation solution.

Xylitol is a natural sugar found in fibrous vegetables and fruits that is used for sweetening tea or coffee and for baking. It is often used by people who want to reduce their sugar intake or by diabetics because it is metabolized in the liver and not by insulin. Xylitol also has the unique property of making it more difficult for bacteria to stick to the nasal and sinus tissues. In addition, most bacteria can't digest xylitol. (Many dentists recommend chewing xylitol chewing gum as a means of preventing cavities, because the bacteria don't stick to the teeth.) Xylitol can be found in most natural food stores or in the diabetic section of the supermarket where it is sold by the pound. It is not sold in pharmacies.

There is a wide range of concentrations that people find useful. In general, I suggest starting with a 1 percent concentration. This is made by adding 2 teaspoons of xylitol to make a 1 percent solution. Add the xylitol along with the saline in Step 2 of the directions on page 54. If a higher concentration is needed, you can gradually increase the concentration by adding three teaspoons of xylitol to make a 1.5 percent solution or four teaspoons to make a 2 percent solution—the best concentration.

The advantage of using xylitol in this manner is that it can be used regularly without concern of building up a resistance to it; it has no side effects; and it costs only about five dollars per pound, so the price is right. Using xylitol in any form, whether eating or irrigating with it, has no effect on producing secondary fungal overgrowth (as many sugars do), and it does not kill the good bacteria in your intestines (as antibiotics do).

In cases of chronic sinusitis, researchers from the University of Pennsylvania found that adding one teaspoon of Johnson's Baby Shampoo to the 16 ounces (500 ml) of saline solution was effective. The baby shampoo contains an ingredient called surfactin, a substance that helps get rid of thick mucus and biofilm. The fact that it is safe for a baby's eyes reflects its safety for use with pulse-wave irrigation in the nose. I generally do not mix the xylitol with the baby shampoo, but use one or the other.

Note: Adding xylitol or baby shampoo to the irrigation solution will seldom cure a stubborn sinus infection. For that you will need to add an antibiotic.

HOW TO ADD MEDICATIONS TO THE PULSE-WAVE IRRIGATOR

To add an antibiotic or any other medication to the nasal irrigator, follow these directions.

1. Add 16 ounces (500 ml) of warm distilled or boiled water to the irrigator basin.

2. Add one packet of Breathe-ease XL or 1 teaspoon of kosher salt with $1/4$ teaspoon of baking soda (to prevent irritation). Mix well.

3. Irrigate 5 ounces (150 ml) through each nostril.

4. Stop and gently clear the nose to allow better contact with the medication.

5. Add the medication to the remaining 6 ounces (200 cc) of saline.

6. Irrigate 3 ounces (100 ml) on each side.

7. After irrigation, remain quietly at the sink for 10 minutes. Don't blow the nose for at least one hour.

PULSE-WAVE IRRIGATION WITH MEDICATIONS
FOR STUBBORN SINUS INFECTIONS

There are situations where the bacteria are well established in the sinuses and an antibiotic may be necessary. For example, for many hospitalized asthmatic patients, a resolution of a sinus infection must take place in order to get the asthmatic well. Stubborn sinus infections can be a complication of any allergy or nasal disorder. Therefore, getting the antibiotic into the sinus cavities for stubborn sinus infections is imperative for sinus, allergy, and asthma health.

Systemic (oral) antibiotics have difficulty reaching into the sinus cavities due to minimal circulation in the nose. It's for this reason that treatment of sinusitis often requires prolonged or repeated courses of antibiotics. An important advantage of using nasal irrigation to deliver the antibiotic is that just as eye drops only affect the eyes, medication by irrigation only affects the nose and sinuses. It bypasses the stomach where it can kill the good bacteria and immune-supportive enzymes.

An important advantage of using pulse-wave irrigation is that it aids in removing biofilm, the thick shield-like coating that develops around the colony of bacteria. This shield is effective in preventing your good white disease-fighting immune cells from attacking the bacteria; it also prevents penetration of the systemic antibiotic. Adding an antibiotic to the irrigation solution gives it a distinct advantage—with a higher concentration, the antibiotics can penetrate the biofilm shield.

Another advantage is that the medication goes directly to where it is needed—to the sinuses. How does the antibiotic enter the sinus cavity? Remember the Bernoulli principle? When the stream that flows past the sinus opening is at a steady pressure and flow, it creates a vacuum that pulls material out of the sinus. When you use this steady stream pulsing action, as the unwanted material is sucked out of the sinus, the pumping action pushes the saline solution into the sinuses. Then the sinuses fill up with the irrigation fluid that contains the medication.

It is important for your doctor to identify the bacterial strain in your sinuses so that the appropriate antibiotic is used. Antibiotics such as gentamycin (Garamycin, Gentak), tobramycin (Tobi, Tobrex), mupirocin (Centany, Bactroban) and amphotericin B (Amphotec, Ambisome) are commonly used; these are all prescription drugs. A major advantage of administering antibiotics this way is that you can use drugs not usually used systemically. Since they are not commonly used, there is much less chance for antibiotic resistance. If your doctor recommends delivering the antibiotic using a nasal irrigator, the directions are often the same as those provided on the previous page.

Adding the antibiotic tobramycin and dexamethasone (Tobradex) to nasal irrigation is a favorite of former ENT surgeon Terence Davidson at the University of California, San Diego, School of Medicine. Tobradex is a combination of an antibiotic and a corticosteroid. Typically, it is found in eye drops and is used to reduce inflammation. Tobradex is available by prescription. Other antibiotics and antifungal additives will be decided by your doctor based on the type of bacteria found on culture from the sinuses and laboratory identification of their sensitivity.

STRENGTHEN IMMUNE FUNCTION

You are born with immunity factors that serve as your body's first line of defense against infection. Good sleep, proper diet, and exercise fortify this defense. You can enhance your immunity by getting regular flu immunizations, eating yogurt, and taking probiotic supplements. Your nasal mucus has immune factors such as immunoglobulins that intercept allergens and other foreign substances and neutralize them. Don't wash out these good immune products from the nose by irrigating three times a day. When the cilia are restored, stop the irrigation. This way you keep the good immune factors in the nose where they belong. To repeat, restoring the cilia is what is important for healing.

6

Is It a Cold, a Sinus Infection, or an Allergy?

How can you prevent a cold during cold season?

- Wash hands thoroughly and regularly with soap.

- Learn how to make Grandma Josephson's chicken soup.

- Keep warm against cold temperatures outside.

- Keep the nasal membranes moist with a moisturizing nasal gel.

- Do your best to get adequate sleep.

- Do your best to stay relaxed.

- Keep your immune system strong with yogurt and probiotics.

- If you have a history of severe cold symptoms, consider daily irrigation.

- Remain on your yacht and avoid contact with sniffers and sneezers. (See if your insurance covers that!)

- Smile.

- Get out of wet clothes as soon as possible.

The common cold is an infection of the nose, sinuses, and respiratory tract caused by a virus. A cold lasts between three and six days. With a cold, pain and swelling are minimal, and there is no green-yellow discharge when it starts. There may be some generalized aching, sneezing, scratchy throat, and runny nose.

Unlike a cold, the signs and symptoms of an allergy are seasonal and follow the pollen calendar. Your nose is stuffy but not painful. You are congested but you don't really feel sick. You can carry on with your daily activities. There is no aching. Your eyes itch and run. The discharge from your nose is often thin and clear. You sneeze excessively at the beginning of the allergy. You have the same symptoms for more than a week and are relieved with most allergy sprays and pills.

Unlike a cold, a sinus infection lasts weeks. You feel quite sick and can't go to work. You blow gobs of green-yellow gunk out of your nose that comes from your sinus cavities. You have a fever and localized pain, you sleep poorly, and many over-the-counter products don't help. You feel better after pulse-wave irrigation. Because the nose, sinuses, and bronchial passages develop from the same embryo layer (the unified airway theory), a bronchial cough with a sinus infection is not unusual. The symptoms blend, manifesting as nasal stuffiness, nasal discharge, coughing, and wheezing, with localized pain in the sinus areas. Therefore, it makes sense to treat every sinus infection as a single body ailment.

HOW DID I "CATCH" A COLD?

Why in the heck are there so many names for the common cold? Is it so that the specialist can sound more authoritative when he says you have acute rhinitis?

Whatever you call it, the common cold is caused by a virus that has multiple forms. There are 200 viruses that cause the common cold. This is why there hasn't been a vaccine developed against the cold virus. A single vaccine for type A would not help you unless you happened to get cold virus type A. Not long ago, one university developed a vaccine for type 23, but the next year the cold virus happened to be type 40 so the vaccine had no beneficial effect. Experience has shown that immunizing for one or two of the common 200 varieties does not immunize against the other varieties of cold viruses.

When you catch a cold, there is usually a one- to three-day incubation period before the symptoms start. If you catch the cold on Sunday, by Tuesday, you will have your symptoms. The reason the virus likes your particular nose is that it thrives at 91°F, which happens to be your nasal temperature. The cold virus can enter your nose via the air or from the virus on your hand or finger that in turn touches your nasal membranes. This is why it is advised to wash your hands frequently during the cold season. Usually, the first sign of a cold is a mild sore throat.

SYMPTOMS OF A COLD

- Chest congestion
- Cough
- Nasal congestion
- Postnasal drainage
- Runny nose
- Sneezing
- Sore throat
- Watery eyes

People catch colds more frequently in winter than in summer because the nasal cilia may slow down in cold weather, so the virus has more opportunity to enter the nose. The air is dry, which enables the cold virus to survive, and close quarters make it easier for the virus to spread. (Do the airlines deliberately plot to seat my patients between two passengers who have colds?) It is estimated that children get as many as six colds a year; adults, as many as three.

The factors that help you resist getting a cold include immunoglobulins, macrophages, and white blood cells. In your nose you have a compound, mentioned earlier, called intracellular adhesion molecule, or ICAM-1. This is the portal of entry of any human cold virus. ICAM-1 is thought to act like a gatekeeper: when the virus enters the nose, the ICAM-1 sends a signal to these immune factors to get here and attack the virus. Once the virus is trapped, the cilia help move it out of the body.

If your immune factors are impaired from lack of sleep or from getting chilled and your cilia are not moving fast, then the cold virus will establish itself in the lining of the nose, where it then begins to multiply. Two days later symptoms begin. Don't panic. Don't rush to the drugstore and buy every pill and spray on the shelf. It is not the end of the world; no one has been hospitalized from catching a cold. The more you relax and follow the WBA, the better for you and everyone exposed to the cold virus around you.

WHY WASH YOUR HANDS DURING AN ACUTE COLD, FLU, OR EBOLA EPIDEMIC?

A virus travels through the air. It may land on the doorknob. When you touch the knob, the virus lands on your hand. Then, without thinking, you touch the inside of your nose. This transfers the virus to your nose where it can enter your body. Even though you honestly swear that you never ever touch your nose, studies show that nearly everyone does this, whether consciously or unconsciously. Therefore, the more you wash your hands with soap, the less chance you have of getting the flu.

A WHOLE BODY APPROACH TO COPING WITH COLDS

In my experience and that of my patients, the WBA can ease the discomfort caused by the symptoms of cold as well as many over-the-counter cold products and pain relievers. At the first sign of a cold, try the following techniques to boost your immune system and keep the virus from multiplying.

KEEP SMILING

Smiling helps prevent a cold. Studies of smiling have demonstrated that putting on a smile during the common cold season reduces the incidence of colds significantly. A smile does two things: First, smiling sends a message to your limbic (stress) system that this is no danger (no tiger), which helps you avoid the negative chemicals that the stress system sends out and which actively reduce your immunity. Second, smiling signals the brain to put out the good chemicals that raise your immune factors. It is the positioning of the facial muscles that does this. Likewise, when the face is paralyzed from trauma or depression, it negatively affects the limbic system.

KEEP THE CILIA MOVING

Tea can boost the body's defense fivefold against disease. A research group at Harvard Medical School reported that five cups of tea a day increases the body's defenses against disease. The immune-activating compound in tea is the amino acid L-theanine. In the liver, L-theanine becomes ethylamine, a molecule that primes the response of an immune blood cell, one of the T cells, which is crucial to the immune response. These T cells, called gamma-delta T cells, prompt the secretion of interferon, a protein produced in response to viral infection that prevents the virus from replicating. Green and black teas are also high in antioxidants and chemically stimulate cilia action.

In my experience, hitting the tea, lemon, and honey as soon as you feel a cold coming on, and going right to bed, is the best preventer and remedy. Warm black or green tea is best, with or without caffeine. Drink eight 8-ounce cups of warm tea with lemon and honey a day. If you drink enough warm tea or chicken soup (see opposite), you may avoid this infection because the cilia wash the virus out.

Research shows that real chicken broth made from whole chickens contains compounds that help break up congestion and eases the flow of nasal secretions. It is also thought to inhibit certain white blood cells that trigger the inflammatory response, which causes sore throats and the production of phlegm. Chicken soup also contains an amino acid called L-cysteine that is released when you make the soup. This amino acid thins mucus in the lungs, aiding in the healing process.

Manuel was in my medical school class. In his second year he felt he knew everything there was to know about medical therapy. He had been taking all the latest products for his cold without any relief. Finally, he went home for school vacation but complained that his grandmother with her old-fashioned non-scientific ideas would probably force him to take chicken soup. When she did feed him the soup, he was completely well the next day. From then on, Manuel put all his patients on chicken soup.

In addition, if you had chicken soup as a child that used to make you well, your brain recalls the good therapy you had with chicken soup, as well as the mothering, and then the brain releases the good chemicals that increase your immune factors. Be sure to make Grandma Josephson's chicken soup.

Which is better? Soup or tea? Frankly, both are good so you can use both.

GRANDMA JOSEPHSON'S HOMEMADE CHICKEN SOUP

3-4 pounds pullet chicken	2 turnips, quartered
1 pound package of chicken wings and giblets	11–12 large carrots, sliced
1 large tomato, cut in half	1 bunch fresh parsley, chopped
3 large yellow onions, quartered	5–6 celery ribs, diced
3 parsnips, quartered	1 bunch fresh dill, chopped
	Salt and pepper to taste

Clean the chicken. Put the chicken in a large pot and cover it with cold water. Bring the water to a boil. Add the wings, giblets, tomato, onions, parsnips, turnips, and carrots. Simmer about $1^1/_2$ hours. Remove the fat from the surface of the broth as it accumulates. Add the parsley, dill, and celery. Cook the soup about 45 minutes longer. Remove the chicken. Put the vegetables in a food processor and process until they are chopped fine or pass through a strainer. Add salt and pepper to taste. Reprinted with permission from Jordan Josephson, M.D. *Sinus Relief Now* (Perigee Trade, 2006). For more information, see www.drjjny.com. Dr. Josephson practices in New York City where colds do cause complications.

GET REST

Get plenty of sleep. When you sleep, your body is repairing itself and helping your immune system to fight off the virus. Allow yourself to nap and do your best to get a sound sleep. If your nose is congested and stuffy, it can interfere with sleep. Inhaling menthol helps and can help make breathing easier. You can use a menthol inhaler such as Vick's vapor inhaler. Another simple way to help the breathing passages remain open while you sleep is to gently adhere a half-inch wide medical-grade tape to the underside of your nose; take the other end of the tape and stretch and secure it to the midline dorsum between the eyes. Gently lift the tip of the nose upward so that it opens the airway.

If your doctor recommends Benadryl (the sedating allergy drug that is also an effective cold remedy) to help you sleep, you get the advantage of having the antihistamine open your nose while you sleep.

REDUCE STRESS AND ANXIETY

The more you relax, the shorter the duration of your cold and the less severe your symptoms will be. Stress and anxiety can complicate every medical condition, whether it is sinus disease, temporomandibular joint dysfunction (TMJ), or the common cold. Honestly, Netflix, the online movie rental service, has cured more colds than Allegra because people get into bed and relax, and let their natural immune systems work. You could also skip the movie and transport yourself to a relaxing island with the visualization exercise below. This exercise combines measured breathing with visualization.

VISUALIZE A TRIP TO A HEALING PLACE

Throughout history mankind has always had places to go to for healing. These places were regularly visited by the sick in body and spirit. Most were characterized by clean air and water, nice temperature, hot springs, and plain food. Most important was the expectation that they would be healed, boosted by the knowledge that other individuals had been cured there. People get better because the hot water, the rest, and the clean air allowed their bodies to regenerate. They also got away from their problems and saw things in a new light. Or they discussed their problems with a wise elder or priest.

Now it's your turn to visit one of these healing places. Be sure to use sight, sound, taste, feel, and smell. Take off your shoes. Sit or lie comfortably. Turn your palms down. Close your eyes. Breathe in for a count of four and out for a count of six. As you exhale, let this be a signal to relax. Picture yourself on a boat or a raft approaching a beautiful island. The water is crystal clear; you can see down to the bottom and see the fish in the water. Try to identify them. As you approach the island, you see hills or mountains green and with all kinds of trees and flowers. You step onto the warm sand; feel the sand. You smell the flowers; recognize the smell. You hear the wind in the trees and so many birds singing. Some of the trees have fruit. You taste the fruit and it is delicious. You feel the coolness of the leaves. Maybe someone has a radio because you hear music as well.

When you feel that you have arrived at this place, turn your palms up. Now you can feel the rays of sun and healing that this place is famous for. You drink the clean water that this island is noted for. You bathe in the healing springs that so many have raved about. And you may wish to speak to some of the counselors about anything that is on your mind. In your mind, picture the counselor and tell him or her of your feelings and concerns. Spend as much time as you wish here. Know that this is another of the healing places that have helped mankind since the beginning of time.

When you are ready for the return trip, put your palms down, get back on the boat or vehicle, and open your eyes. Physiologically, if I were to measure you, I would find that some healing has actually taken place!

When you do this visualization, you change your body chemistry. In the healing place your stomach is not in spasm, your neck is not tight, your elevated blood pressure is reduced, and your stress chemicals are lowered. Healing takes place.

USE PULSE-WAVE IRRIGATION IF NEEDED

For my patients who get very sick when they get a cold, I have them use the pulse-wave irrigation to wash the ICAM-1 from the nose. When you use pulse-wave irrigation after exposure to everyone in the office who is sneezing and coughing, this helps you to avoid the cold infection. When the ICAM-1 is removed, there is no portal of entry for the cold virus to enter the body. This can be beneficial to people with a history of frequent winter colds that result in absence from work.

Generally, I do not recommend nasal irrigation to treat a cold. Most colds are limited and are well controlled by the measures previously discussed.

If you have a history of severe cold symptoms, ask your doctor if using a pulse-wave irrigator during the cold season to remove ICAM-1 and increase cilia movement is recommended for you.

Since ICAM-1 is the portal of entry of the cold virus, I often have patients "block" the portal of entry by covering the nasal areas with Breathe-ease XL Nasal Moisturizing Gel so that the cold virus can't enter. This is good medicine when everyone in the office has a cold and is sneezing and coughing. I recommend it for my patients who get sick when they fly.

OTHER HELPFUL HINTS FOR SNUFFING OUT A COLD

- If your blow your nose, remember to do it gently. By not blowing hard when your nose is stuffed with lots of thick mucus, you can prevent much serious damage to your nasal passageways and ears. Sounds simple, but gentle nose blowing can make a world of difference in the way that your cold progresses.

- If you sneeze, also do it gently so you don't spread germs.

- The drier your nose, the more chance for a cold virus to enter. Use a nasal moisturizing gel like Breathe-ease XL to coat the nasal passages.

- Don't get chilled. Keep warm against the cold. If your clothes get wet outdoors, change them as soon as possible.

- Skip the heavily advertised zinc products. Evidence indicates that they may shorten the cold somewhat, but they don't affect the severity of the cold—and there are side effects. Zinc nasal spray has now been banned by the FDA because of so many reports of anosmia (loss of smell, see Chapter 12). This is not surprising since it is standard research practice to use dilute zinc sulfate spray to deaden the smell sense in research animal studies. Also, echinacea root and juice extracts are a commonly used herbal treatment for infection. A recent study reported that the herb echinacea did not help symptoms of a cold in children.

- Flying during the cold season is difficult. My patients benefit by carrying tea bags on the plane so they can drink lots of tea, and by using a nasal moisturizing gel such as Breathe-ease XL to coat the nose. The nasal gel can be applied into the nose the morning of the flight and then used every three hours during the flight. This acts as a cover to prevent the virus from entering the nasal tissue. The tea provides L-theanine for immunity and keeps the cilia moving.

COMPLICATIONS FROM THE COMMON COLD

If treated promptly with the WBA, most colds will clear up quickly. It is important to count how many colds you get a year. If it is one cold a year, I don't think that trying to reduce that with medication is of value. Generally, people who get one cold a year at age thirty have them much less frequently as they age. If you get one a year without complications, you are fortunate.

The patients I see get colds frequently and are seeking relief. In addition to relieving their cold symptoms, I work on building up their poor resistance. Eating yogurt and taking probiotic supplements are two preventatives I always recommend for raising immunity. Smiling is a definite aid since it reduces the stress chemicals that lower immunity.

If a person's overall immunity is poor, a cold may linger past six days with cough and aching. This often means that a secondary bacterial infection is present and a doctor should be consulted.

And what if your doctor cultures your nose and you have a bacterial infection? What if he or she prescribes an antibiotic? Should you take it? Repeatedly, you hear that you should reduce the overuse of antibiotics. For some patients, a trial of the WBA might be enough to ward off the need for the antibiotic. It is not possible to predict when the remedies might be effective. I do know that many times I have prescribed antibiotics and next visit the patient was fine, even though the prescription was never filled. Was this because of the patient's determination to get well without resorting to pills? Or was this the result of the WBA?

PART TWO

COMMON ALLERGY AND SINUS-RELATED COMPLAINTS

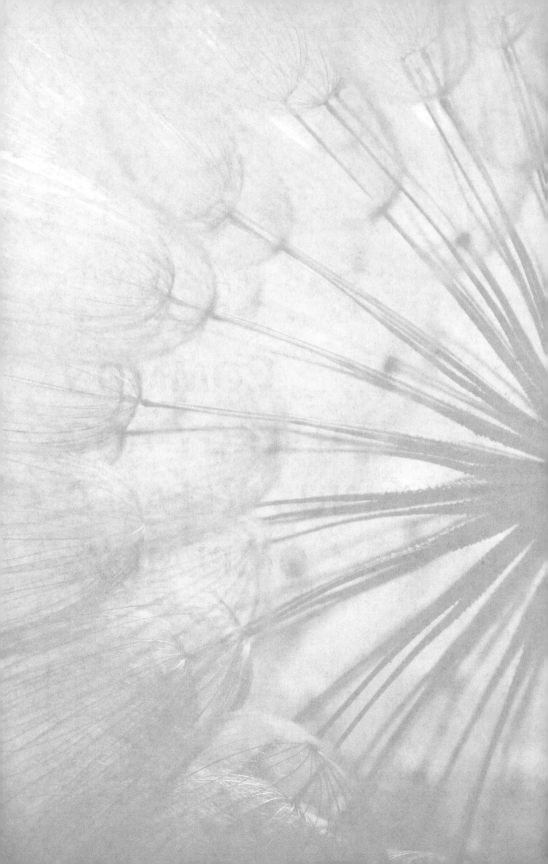

7

Is It a Sinus Headache, a Tension Headache, or a Migraine?

DOES THIS SOUND LIKE YOU?

- Daily head pains.
- Daily pounding head pain with visual disturbance.
- Head pain severe enough to keep you from daily activity.
- Headache associated with nausea and vomiting.

- Headaches that keep you bedridden in a dark room.
- Severe headaches partially relieved by walking about.
- Headaches that start in the neck and end in the sinuses.

If you are one of the 50 million people with these symptoms, I have some suggestions for you. There are some simple steps that anyone can take to prevent or relieve headaches. This is because headaches have multiple triggers and eliminating some of them can reduce the frequency of headaches or may even eliminate them.

SINUS AND OTHER COMMON HEADACHES

When a new patient comes to my office, the most common sinus complaint is headache. Because the sinus cavities are located above the eyes, between the eyes, and below the eyes, the pain from them may be felt in many areas of the face and head. Your pain may be one-sided, like a pressure, above the eye, due to sinusitis. You may have pain in the front of your head that is like a heavy pressure due to sinusitis. You may have pain in your left upper jaw that is sinusitis. Unfortunately, head pain can come from many other factors because nerves to the head connect to other nerves. And what feels like a sinus headache may actually be a migraine, a tension headache, or one of the following kinds of headache. Headaches are easy to misdiagnose. Becoming familiar with other types of head pain that can mimic a sinus headache will help you differentiate a real sinus headache from among them.

SINUS HEADACHES

Sinus headaches are associated with a swelling of the membranes lining the sinus cavities. Most pain from sinusitis occurs within the sinuses—the result of air, pus, and mucus being trapped within the obstructed sinuses. With sinus infection, there is inflammation including swelling. That is the pain of sinus headache. The greater the sinus drainage is blocked, the more painful the sinus headache.

Pain above the eye may be from the frontal sinus. Pressure above the eye socket and pain at the roof of the eye socket indicate frontal sinusitis. This is because the floor of the frontal sinus is the roof of the eye socket. The eye may be swollen and looking up or down may be painful. Pain in the frontal sinus area may also be due to referred pain from the neck.

Pain below the eye is associated with the large maxillary sinus. Maxillary sinus pain may involve the inferior alveolar nerve that serves the floor of the maxillary sinus and the teeth of the upper jaw. Dental infections can drain into the maxillary sinus or teeth can press on that nerve. Sometimes both a dentist and an ENT doctor need to be consulted when the pain is in the cheek. (For an illustration of an infection in the maxillary sinus, see the web link in the Resources section.) If this pain is not combined with nasal congestion, it suggests a dental origin.

Pain in the upper cheeks, in the nose, and between the eyes indicates an ethmoid sinus pain. This is also accompanied by nasal congestion. Moving the eyes from side to side may be painful and one eye may lag behind the other eye.

Pain from the sphenoid sinus is highly variable and vague. Sometimes patients have difficulty expressing this pain as being at the top of the head or between the eyes.

SYMPTOMS OF A SINUS HEADACHE

- Pain intensified by bending forward, lying down, or shaking the head.
- Same pain for weeks.
- Location between the eyes.
- Location above the upper teeth.
- May be uncomfortable to chew.
- In the maxillary sinus it is difficult to tell if it is tooth or cheek.
- Pressing on the pain area is painful.
- In the frontal sinus, pressing the floor of the sinus (roof of the eye socket) is painful.
- Pain made worse by migraine medications.

Sinus headaches are not pounding or pulsating. Usually there is a complaint of nasal congestion or discharge. Sinus headaches tend to worsen as you bend forward or lie down. Sinus headaches are long lasting and present for days to weeks. In general, however, sinus headaches are not severe. Over-the-counter products such as aspirin (Bayer, Ecotrin), ibuprofen (Advil, Motrin), and acetaminophen (Tylenol) are normally effective at relieving the pain. Later in the chapter, I'll discuss other remedies for coping with sinus headaches.

VACUUM HEADACHES

A vacuum sinus headache is very painful. The reason a vacuum headache is so painful is that it starts at 33,000 feet where the atmospheric pressure is low. It is not unusual at this pressure for the nose to clog up and for the sinuses to become blocked, especially if the cabin air is dry and your fluid intake is low. Because the sinuses are blocked, upon landing, the pressure within the sinuses remains low, while the air pressure outside the body and sinuses is now higher. This creates a type of vacuum effect with the pressure inside the sinuses at about 10 pounds per square inch (psi) and outside pressure of 15 pounds psi. The resulting head pain is similar to having a five-pound weight pressing on your nerves. Scuba diving can also trigger a vacuum headache. Fortunately, the pain is eased as soon as the sinus blockage is relieved. Then, the air enters and the vacuum is relieved. The relief is like having a five-pound weight removed from your eye.

If the diagnosis is a vacuum headache, opening the blockage in order to equalize the pressure inside the sinus cavity is the preferred treatment. Using oxymetazoline (Neo-Synephrine Extra-Strength nasal deconges-tant spray) with 1 percent phenylephrine, or Benzedrex, a nasal decon-gestant spray, may open the blockage. Your doctor may also choose to place a pledget (cotton strip) soaked in Neo-Synephrine Extra-Strength spray against the sinus opening to open it. Breathing helium will pene-trate through the smallest openings to relieve the vacuum. The prote-olytic enzymes papain (from papaya) and bromelain (from pineapple) work to help open and keep the sinus doorways open (for more on these enzymes, see page 117).

HEADACHE PAIN ON A SCALE OF 1–10

HEADACHE TYPE	LOCATION	DURATION	PAIN SCALE*
Sinus headache	Sinus areas	Present for days	2–3
Tension headache	Back of neck and above eyes	Present for weeks	2–3
Premenstrual headache	Generalized, entire head	Starts 10 days before menstruation	2–3
Migraine headache	Usually one-sided	Typically lasts several hours	6–8
Trigeminal neuralgia headache	Well localized to area of nerve distribution	Is longer lasting than a cluster headache	9–10
Cluster headache	Entire head hurts	Presents for an hour or less	10

*Note: Scale is from 1 (lowest level) of pain to 10 (highest level).

TENSION HEADACHES

Tension headaches are the most common type of headache. It is estimated that about 90 percent of all headaches are tension headaches. Tension headaches, as the term suggests, are caused by muscular tension.

A common cause of muscular tension and tension headaches is bad posture. Hours in front of a computer causes headache from the neck muscles being strained. Following a whiplash injury, there is headache due to trauma of the posterior neck muscles. Stress is another common cause of tension headaches. Being stressed causes a fight-or-flight reaction in the body with a tightening of neck muscles.

For my patients with tension headaches, I recommend physical therapy. I find that the physical therapists do a good job of diagnosing and treating muscles, whether to make them stronger or to reduce spasm or tightness. I also recommend all tension headache sufferers do the cervical shower exercise for the circulation for four minutes daily (see page 114). It's one of the best and simplest ways for easing muscle tension and making the blood vessels less "irritable."

Because posture is extremely important, whenever possible, use a full-length mirror to check your posture. When you are shopping, check yourself in the store windows as you pass. Camille's parents tried everything to get their teenage daughter to have good posture. Finally, her brother Dan put a mirror by Camille's computer and then she sat up straight.

Although there are medications for headache, physical therapy, shower massage, measured breathing and muscle relaxation (see page 50), and good posture can be crucial to preventing a headache. Keeping a headache diary (see page 111) can also help.

PHYSICAL THERAPY TO RELIEVE HEADACHES

Headache patients do better on an exercise program and sometimes the right series of exercises can be the "cure." I make sure that my patients engage in an exercise program, whether to reduce stress or to improve circulation or muscle action. I frequently refer patients to physical therapists in order to have them prescribe an

individualized program. One patient had certain neck muscles that needed strengthening. Another hated exercise because he couldn't do 100 pushups; in other words,
he was trying to do precisely the wrong types of exercise! When he followed the individual program prescribed for him, he did fine.

Walking is always a good to do. I recommend that if you don't already have a
dog, find one in the neighborhood and borrow one to take walking.

In any illness, the patient benefits when he or she assumes responsibility for his
or her health. At the end of a recent international conference on obesity, the doctors
complained, "For three days all they talked about was diet pills and their dangerous
side effects. Nobody said anything about exercise, nutrition, and good habits!" No
wonder we need the WBA here!

MIGRAINE HEADACHES

A migraine has unique characteristics that distinguish it from other kinds
of headaches. A migraine headache generally comes from the blood vessels becoming twitchy or spastic. In many cases, it starts with an aura of
flashing lights, a feeling of lightheadedness, a need to urinate, and a
knowing, or premonition, called a prodromata, that the headache is coming. The aura occurs when the blood vessels constrict. Then, as the blood
vessels slam open, they often causing leakage through the vessel walls;
this is the cause of the headache pain. The pain is usually described as
intense and throbbing, and it can occur on one or both sides of the
head. In addition to the pain, a migraine headache may be accompanied
by nausea, vomiting, and sensitivity to light, sound, and movement. The
pain is more severe than a tension headache, and the patient feels better lying down in a dark room. If the patient awakens in the middle of
the night with a throbbing severe headache, this is diagnostic of a
migraine. On average, a migraine may occur twice a week and last several hours; there is huge variation however.

Melissa had a migraine five times in January, but hasn't had any since.

Mark continues to get a bad migraine headache twice a week despite
getting treatment.

There is both a hormonal and familial relationship in migraine. In families where one sister began taking birth control pills and then started to get migraines, another sister got the same result when she started the contraceptive. Migraines may stop or increase in pregnancy or menopause. Some women have been known to have numerous pregnancies because they were free of migraine headaches then. Children can get migraines, too. Throughout history many people have become addicted to narcotic drugs because of their migraines.

For my patients with migraine, I have them focus a shower stream to the back of the neck for several minutes, while slowly and gently rotating the head from side to side. This action helps train the blood vessels not to be so twitchy. Some people can take 125 milligrams (mg) of slow-release niacin (vitamin B3), twice a day, without getting the headache. This maintains the blood vessels in a dilated state so that when the trigger comes on, the vessels can't constrict much because they are already open, and they can't quite slam open so vigorously because they are dilated. A migraine won't respond to aspirin (Bayer), acetaminophen (Tylenol), ibuprofen (Advil), naproxen (Aleve) or other over-the-counter pain relievers—if it does, it may not be a migraine. Excedrin Migraine, another over-the-counter pain reliever, works for some migraine sufferers; it contains 250 mg of acetaminophen, 250 mg of aspirin, and 65 mg of caffeine.

Some choices for relief of a migraine headache that require a prescription include sumatriptan (Imitrex), zolmitriptan (Zomig), rizatriptan (Maxalt), and naratriptan (Amerge), as well as dihydroergotamine (Migranal) nasal spray.

For migraine headaches that occur three or more times a month, preventive treatment is often recommended. Strangely, medications used for heart conditions are often effective for preventing migraines. The current ones recommended by the American Academy of Neurology and the American Headache Society include: acetazolamide (Diamox), a diuretic for glaucoma and congestive heart failure; lisinopril (Zestril), an angiotensin-converting enzyme (ACE) inhibitor that helps to lower blood pressure; methysergide (Sansert), a weak constrictor of blood vessels; and propranolol (Inderal), a beta-blocker that treats hypertension. Butterbur (*Petasites hybridus*), an herb used primarily for allergy, helps to reduce spasms and inflammation. Another herb, hibiscus (*Hibiscus sabdariffa*), has antispasmodic and antihypertensive properties and contains the same chemicals as Zestril and Diamox. For a recipe for hibiscus tea, see below.

Other medications sometimes used as preventives include amitriptyline (Elavil), an antidepressant; gabapentin (Neurontin), an anti-epileptic medication; valproic acid (Depakote), an anticonvulsant; and venlafaxine (Effexor), an anti-anxiety drug. Dozens of foods and beverages can trigger migraines and other headaches, but most people are bothered by only a few. For help on how to identify the foods that may affect you, see page 111.

Occasionally, a migraine can follow a blow to the head. A patient sustained a blow from a shelf that fell on her head and she had had headaches for a year without relief from any therapies. After a careful history and evaluation, these turned out to be migraines, and she responded immediately to treatment with Imitrex. Why did she develop true migraine despite having a typical "simple" head trauma? The mechanism for this is not understood, but developing migraine after a work injury is a common reason for therapies not being effective.

HIBISCUS TEA: A NATURAL MIGRAINE PREVENTIVE

Zestril and Diamox are two drugs that are recommended for migraine prevention. In one study, hibiscus tea acted the same as Zestril for reducing blood pressure and it also has a diuretic effect like Diamox. Since hibiscus tea has the same properties as the two products recommended for migraine prevention, why not take the tea instead for migraine prevention? My friend Dora says it prevents her migraine. Here is her recipe for hibiscus tea:

2 cups dry hibiscus (also known as Jamaica flowers or flor de Jamaica)

6 cups water

$3/4$ cup granulated sugar (more if desired)

Mint leaves (optional)

ice

Rinse and drain the dried hibiscus. Bring the water to a boil in a medium-size pot. Add the hibiscus and sugar and stir continuously while the mixture boils for one minute. Be careful not to boil the tea too long or it will have a slightly bitter after-taste. Remove from the heat and steep for two hours. Let the tea cool, and then strain it into a pitcher. Refrigerate until time to serve. Ladle into a tall glass filled with ice and garnish with fresh mint leaves if desired.

LESS COMMON TYPES OF HEADACHES

There are other types of headaches that can cause pain in the region of the sinuses, but they are less common than tension headaches, migraines, or sinus headaches.

CIRCULATION (VASCULAR) HEADACHES

Blood vessels open and close. Sometimes this expansion and contraction occurs with great force, causing the vessels to slam open and shut. This is characteristic of vascular headaches. If you apply ice to the back of your neck, and then apply heat, you will get a headache. In a migraine headache, discussed above, this mechanism causes extreme vasoconstriction followed by extreme vasodilation. In some instances, a circulation headache can develop into a migraine headache.

Nellie was taking scuba lessons. She was wearing a wet suit for the cold water at a 100-foot depth. When she surfaced, she sat with the bright sun heating the back of her neck to warm her cold neck. She got this terrible headache and the instructor thought she might have bends. This condition occurs when a diver decompresses too quickly, which causes gas bubbles to form in the bloodstream. These bubbles can block tiny blood vessels and lead to joint pain, tiredness, headache, and in extreme cases stroke and death. She was rushed into a decompression chamber. I met her at the emergency station and diagnosed a vascular headache instead, which easily responded to treatment. Knowing the mechanism, Nellie could continue her scuba activities.

All headache sufferers should do the cervical shower exercise for the circulation (see page 114). It's one of the best and simplest ways for easing muscle tension and making the blood vessels less irritable. Cold shrinks blood vessels and heat expands them. Therefore, wear a scarf when you go to a movie in case you need to keep your neck warm, and never drive at night with the wind blowing on your neck. Many of my patients respond to small doses of slow-release vasodilators such as niacin to keep the blood vessels open in order to avoid the constriction. On the other hand, niacin may bring on a headache by vasodilation in some patients.

If a migraine is one-sided, for example on the right side of the head, icing the right side of the face in front of the jaw joint may stop a migraine headache from developing. Incidentally, never drive at night with the cold wind blowing directly on your cheek. This can chill your facial nerve and result in facial paralysis!

CLUSTER HEADACHES

Another type of headache is the cluster headache. Also known as a histamine headache and Horton's headache, this type of headache is episodic; meaning that it can come in bunches—say three a week for five weeks, and then not return for many months. The pain is severe (a ten on any scale) and may be accompanied by ptosis (a droopy upper eyelid), miosis (a constricted pupil), tearing or redness of the conjunctiva, and a runny nose—symptoms that are linked to the autonomic nervous system. The pain is described as boring (piercing) and is typically concentrated behind or above the eye; it is one-sided only and repeats on that side.

Cluster headaches do not appear to be related to hormones, age, or stress. They tend to occur in middle-aged men. Typically, they last less than thirty minutes and may repeat over a twenty-four-hour period or longer, occurring even while you sleep. Once the cluster is over, the area affected is sore for some time.

Treatments include breathing 100 percent oxygen though a mask, using migraine medications, and drinking very strong coffee. I have had success with these headaches by injecting triamcinolone acetonide (Kenalog) into the inferior (lower) turbinate in the nose.

FOOD-RELATED HEADACHES

Food allergies can cause headaches in addition to such gastrointestinal symptoms as an itching mouth, lips, and tongue; difficulty in swallowing; nausea; and stomach cramps. Food allergy may be the regular reaction of IgE to products that the body thinks are harmful or it could be an overreaction to certain otherwise harmless products. People who suffer from frequent headaches may be reacting to certain foods to which they are allergic or sensitive. Celiac disease is an example of an immune reaction to the protein gluten in wheat and similar products.

Try keeping a headache diary (see below). You can do a simple self-test to determine whether a food is a cause. Try two weeks without the suspect food and then reintroduce the food and eat lots of it for a week. If you get a headache after consuming the substance, eliminate it permanently from your diet. (The most common suspect foods are listed below.) Niacin is a vasodilator and in some people may cause headaches. Check the label of your multivitamin, if the formula contains niacin that could be a trigger, too.

A HEADACHE DIARY

By recording when a headache comes on, sometimes the answer to what is causing your headache becomes quite obvious. The diary may show that the headache comes on premenstrually or after eating at the Mexican restaurant or when driving the convertible with the top down on a sunny day. Foods can trigger headaches. The diary can tell you if the preservative in dried cherries was followed by a headache.

Lisa wondered why, when she ate Italian at home, she experienced no headache. But on a date to an Italian restaurant, she got a headache. It turns out that the culprit was the red wine at the restaurant. Red wine is a very common headache trigger, not only for migraine but also for simple headaches as well.

The diary will immediately diagnose a headache from monosodium glutamate (MSG), migraine from red wine, and headache from visits by the mother-in-law. To identify the foods that affect you, avoid the most common potential triggers for two weeks:

- Alcoholic beverages, including cooking sherry, and especially red wine

- Artificial sweeteners, including those found in diet sodas

- Beans, including lima, string, garbanzo, and lentils

- Cheeses, except for American, ricotta, cottage, Velveeta, and cream cheese

- Chocolate, carob, and licorice

- Bacon and all canned, cured, or processed meat products containing sulfites

- Mustard (non-dry), ketchup, and mayonnaise

- Pickles, chili peppers, and olives

- Soy sauce, olive oil, and vinegar, except for white and apple cider

- Whole milk, sour cream, buttermilk, whipped cream, and ice cream

After the two-week period, resume eating one food from the prohibited list per week. If you experience no change, the food is not a headache trigger for you. Record this information in the diary. If your headaches return or worsen, the reintroduced food is probably a trigger and should be permanently eliminated from your diet. If a particular product brings on your migraine headache, it doesn't mean you are allergic to it. It is not a typical IgE-histamine type 1 allergy and will not react to skin or blood testing. The reaction is different from a histamine reaction and is more of a chemical/hormonal response. This information can assist your doctor in treating you.

Note: See *The Headache Prevention Cookbook* (2000) by David Marks, M.D., and Laura Marks, M.D., for more information.

NECK (CERVICAL) HEADACHES

A cervical headache is caused by referred pain from the neck. If your computer screen is positioned too low or if the contrast and brightness of the screen is poor, you can strain your neck and trigger a headache. If your desk chair is so low so that you have to strain your neck to see your computer, it could trigger a headache. A chair that is too soft can also trigger a headache. As a rule, the softer the chair, the worse it is for the headache patient (as well as for the back patient). One of the newer ergonomic chairs may be best for you. Check the lighting at your desk, too.

My friend was upset. Since he moved into his new office with a fabulous view of the river, two of his secretaries had developed headaches. When I inquired about some of these common office triggers, the answer was simple: in order to enjoy the view, his staff had positioned their desks and computers so they could see the river. The glare from the water caused them to squint and strain. Instead of pills, the solution was to turn the desks around.

Andrew had been my patient for years. He had recently developed bad headaches and his primary doctor had referred him to a neurologist. After all kinds of tests, he was given a prescription for pain pills. He came to me hoping I could find a solution. He had cervical muscle spasms. I asked if he was somehow straining his neck. No, not really, he explained, except that sometimes he had trouble looking over the hood of his new low slung sports car. Turns out that sitting too low while driving and straining to see over the car hood, strained his muscles and caused his headache. The cure was a five-dollar seat cushion! His car seat was too low and he had to strain to see the road. Andrew wondered what to do with all the prescribed pain pills he didn't need anymore.

PAIN REFERRED TO THE HEAD FROM THE NECK

A patient presents with a history of recurrent frontal sinus pain. On examination the nose looks fine; the CT scan is clear. When the neck is palpated, the frontal sinus area, above the eyes, is painful. This is because the nerve root of the trigeminal nerve that supplies sensation to the frontal area gets stimulated when certain cervical roots from the neck are painful. Palpating the neck and noting the tightness and spasm there makes the diagnosis. Treatment here is to treat the neck. The right type of massage may be the cure. If this sounds like you, do the shower massage and cervical neck massage daily (see page 114). Any sprained muscle can result in pain, and if it is referred to the skull, it is felt in the head as a headache. This referred pain is seen often and causes a lot of unnecessary X-rays and medication.

David watched his health, exercise, and diet. Yet he kept getting these dull headaches while playing bridge or a game on the computer. He needed a diagnosis because a new job required more computer screen time and he didn't know if he could do it. When I palpated his neck, the left muscle mass was distinctly less than on the right side. He had had a mild case of polio as a child that left the neck muscles on the left weak. Physical therapy healed the problem by building up the strength of the weak muscles and improving his posture. (Before polio vaccination many persons had mild cases and were not even aware they had polio. However, even these mild cases can leave certain muscles weak. These weak muscles can get weaker as the patient ages.)

MASSAGE FOR RELAXING TENSE MUSCLES

The best way to avoid headaches is to avoid muscle tension. To help cramped muscles, do the following massage-type cervical exercises. Both work well for preventing and treating headaches.

Take a hot shower at night before bedtime. Stand with your back to the showerhead and focus the water stream on the back of the neck. Slowly and gently turn the head from side to side as if you are trying to see who is standing behind you. Do this for four minutes. This removes lactic acid buildup (a byproduct of muscle strain that cause soreness) and makes the blood vessels less "irritable."

In addition, try massaging the neck with a menthol gel or ointment like Tiger's Balm. The massage should be done using a milking movement to push the lactic acid and inflammatory factors out of the muscles in the direction of the lymphatic and venous flow towards the heart. This moves the accumulated fluids in the direction of lymphatic flow and is best for removing accumulated lactic acid and other unwanted residue.

New studies show that any sore muscle that gets proper massage therapy is improved. The overused muscle contains specific inflammatory chemicals. If it is the neck, massaging the muscle towards the heart will remove them. Actually, the entire body feels better by reduction of those chemicals. This is why everyone feels better after they get a massage.

Caution: Never crack the neck unless an MRI or CT scan shows that it is safe to do so. In France it is illegal to perform neck cracking without a previous MRI evaluation. Forcibly turning a "frozen" neck to one side can splinter bones that sever the spinal cord.

PREMENSTRUAL HEADACHES

Headaches that typically begin ten days before menstruation are usually due to water retention and fluctuating levels of estrogen and progesterone. Headache specialist and physician Lee Kudrow has found that eating dark chocolate, which is rich in a natural trace amine called phenylethylamine, also stops these headaches, if taken ten days before the onset of menses. The cocoa powder that you add to milk is also effective. Diuretics taken ten days before menstruation are also effective. By eliminating salt fifteen days before the onset of menstruation and drinking distilled water, patients are often relieved of premenstrual headaches thanks to the diuretic effect of lowered salt intake. The distilled water has no salt and pulls salt and water out of the body.

Birth control pills that are high in estrogen are associated with headaches. For some women, starting birth control pills can bring on migraine headaches. This occurred in one patient and her sister developed migraine headaches too when she began the contraceptive pills. Contraceptives low in estrogen and primarily in progesterone have lower headache results.

RHINOGENIC HEADACHES

Nasal tissue may swell in the presence of an allergy or an infection and cause head pressure that occasionally is painful. In a rhinogenic headache, contact caused by swelling of the nasal and sinus tissues can result in headache or facial pain without inflammation or infection or allergy. For example, the nasal septum (the wall dividing the nasal cavity into halves) may be severely deviated so that the slightest swelling pushes the nasal tissue into this septum tissue and causes pain, much like sticking a pin into the nasal membrane. In such patients, the septum is almost touching or is actually touching one of the turbinates. If I anesthetize that area and the pain goes away, that makes the diagnosis. To prevent further headaches of this type, straightening the deviated septum surgically so that it no longer touches the nasal tissues will correct the problem. Rhinogenic headaches are usually constant, not throbbing, and are controlled with non-steroidal medications such as naproxen (Naprosyn).

Occasionally, the two nasal bones are separated at the bridge of the nose. Here, cold wind can affect the nasal chamber and cause pain. Therefore, headaches while skiing occur when the nasal bones are not joined at the top.

Temporomandibular Joint Disorder Headaches (TMJ)

Facial pain, pain in the temples, or pain above the ear arising from temporomandibular joint disorder is called a TMJ headache. This common type of headache is caused by a misalignment or damage to the temporomandibular joint, the hinge-like joint that connects the jawbone to the sides of the skull. Injury to this joint can be caused by stress and the fight-or-flight response, in which the jaw tightens in response to a perceived threat or in readiness for actual combat; by a severe dental problem that causes the muscles of the jaw to be unbalanced; by grinding the teeth at night (bruxism); or by a combination of issues involving the jaw joint and muscles that control jaw movement. The resulting TMJ pain may be referred to the neck, skull, and sinus areas. The pain is constant, not pulsing, and is relieved by aspirin.

To diagnose TMJ, put your fingers just in front of the ear canals. Feel the bones move as you open your jaw wide repeatedly. Is there an audible sound? Can you feel grating and noise? If you do, that means the pain from the TMJ may be causing your headache. Now draw a vertical line on your mirror. Open your jaw by lining up your face to the vertical line. Does the jaw open to the side? Is there a severe deviation? If an ENT doctor finds that the jaw opens to the side, he or she can take electromagnetic measurements to determine which muscle is pulling excessively and which is weaker.

I have my patients practice learning to open their jaw on the midline by looking in a mirror. Use measured breathing—breathing in for a count or four and out for a count of six—and relax your jaw when you relax on the exhalation. You don't open the jaw; you relax it so that it opens by gravity. This allows the muscles to balance. When the jaw opens to the side, it means that the jaw muscles are not balanced, and this is the cause of the TMJ pain. Dentists prescribe night guards for this problem. For my patients who have failed to relieve their TMJ headaches with a night guard, the mirror feedback and breathing exercise on page 152 has worked well. (Draw a vertical line on the mirror and relax the jaw as in action #5.) Once the jaw muscles are balanced, that should relieve the problem.

With pain, there is usually inflammation. In severe cases, you can use a bandana or an Ace bandage to support the jaw from the scalp and to rest the jaw; also avoid chewing. Most over-the-counter anti-inflammatories such as Naprosyn help. My product Clear-ease is a combination of papain from papaya and bromelain from pineapple. You melt the lozenge in your mouth between the cheek and gum. These proteolytic enzymes work to reduce the inflammation. I recommend one lozenge, four times a day. (For more on these enzymes, see below.)

WHAT ARE PROTEOLYTIC ENZYMES?

Proteolytic enzymes are substances that break down proteins. They weaken tough muscle fibers and are used in cooking to soften meat. Enzymes are also used as a treatment to thin mucus and reduce swelling. They can be great for resolving problems like thick mucus and difficulty clearing your stuffed up ears, and for any kind of bruise (boxers like them). They can be very effective and are quite safe—as long as you are not allergic to them or to the plant they are derived from—but you have to be careful about where you get them from and how you use them.

A good proteolytic enzyme formula is a bromelain and papain preparation that has calibrated enzyme activity. Many commercial enzyme preparations have enzyme activity so low that they do no good. Many are also made to be chewed or swallowed, which often has little effect, because the enzymes are inactivated by stomach acids. For these reasons, buy proteolytic enzymes that have calibrated enzyme activity and dissolve them between your cheek and gum.

Trigeminal Neuralgia Headaches

The pain from a trigeminal neuralgia headache comes from the trigeminal nerve, the fifth cranial nerve. This nerve transmits the feelings of touch and pain from the face, eyes, sinuses, and mouth to the brain. It has three parts and roots: the frontal part, the maxillary part, and the lower jaw area. When the pain is referred from the neck, it usually refers to the upper frontal division of the trigeminal nerve, above the eyes. This is because, in the spinal cord, the nerve roots reverse and the root of the trigeminal nerve lies next to the root of the cervical nerves. Trigeminal neuralgia is an extremely severe nerve disorder that causes a stabbing or electric shock-like pain in parts of the face. The pain is usually only on one side of the face, often around the eyes, cheek, and lower part of the face, and may last a few seconds or minutes but can become continuous. Pain from the trigeminal nerve can come from a viral infection and requires good care. I refer these patients to a neurologist who deals with these headaches all the time. This severe neuralgia is not helped by relaxation or stress reduction. Trigeminal neuralgias can be caused by aneurysms, bony thickening in canals (bone spurs), and tissue growths that press on the nerve. Note: The area above the eye socket may be the area of trigeminal neuralgic pain. Here, the supraorbital nerve from the first division of the trigeminal nerve exits through the bone. Massaging this area would make the nerve swell and increase trigeminal pain.

Vision-Related Headaches

If your vision correction is off, it can trigger a headache because the eyes and other muscles squeeze in order to focus. Thus, if your headaches come on after reading, check your eyeglass or contact prescription. Squinting does the same thing. Nearly everyone gets a headache when he or she first starts wearing bifocals, but that is temporary.

Victor was a forty-eight-year-old accountant who came to me for sinus headaches. He had been diagnosed with headaches due to stress on the job and had a prescription for pain pills to take four times a day. I noticed him squinting and having trouble filling out the patient information sheet. The diagnosis? He needed reading glasses, and not pain pills. Stress? Yes, he was stressed at having trouble reading the numbers, but that all cleared when he purchased the cheap reading glasses at the discount store.

I see headaches from daytime driving in people who wear transitional glasses that automatically darken in the sun. But these lenses don't darken inside a car no matter how bright the glare. Inside a car, the transitional lenses don't work, and sunglasses are needed for daytime driving. These sun-glare headaches are usually short in duration, whereas the neck-strain headaches last all day.

DIAGNOSING A SINUS HEADACHE

Unfortunately, the nerves of the head can refer to various parts of the body. For example, pain in the frontal sinus area should be from the frontal sinuses, but in practice it can be due to cervical pain, a migraine, neuralgia, or even from a different sinus. As you can see, correct diagnosis may be difficult.

Julie came to me referred by a friend. I was the third doctor she was seeing for her sinus headache. She came with a bag of medications—sprays, pills, and herbs. She complained that she continued to have sinus headaches despite "spending a fortune" on treatments. Her headache was maxillary; meaning that the pain was below her eyes in the cheek area. It was sometimes on both sides or could be either right or left. A dentist ruled out any dental problem and a CT scan of her sinuses showed no inflammation. Nasal cultures were negative for any significant bacteria that would indicate an infection.

Her medical history revealed one clue: her headaches usually were worse about two in the afternoon. I quickly located an area in her neck that was the trigger for her headaches. An MRI showed cervical pathology. Her headaches were cervical. Usually pain from the neck is referred to the first division of the trigeminal nerve, to the area above the eyes. In Julie's case, her cervical nerves referred to the second division of the trigeminal nerve, which is the area under her eyes in the cheek area.

Trudy sought relief from her sinus headaches. These awakened her in the middle of the night. They were always on the right side but none of the prescribed medicines were helping her. She was afraid to go to sleep for fear of another headache. Headaches that wake you up out of a sound sleep and are severe are almost always migraines. Trudy responded to migraine therapy.

In general, if the head pain is above the eye and that area is tender, this suggests a sinus headache caused by frontal sinusitis. Commonly, it is referred pain from the muscles in the back of the neck.

If the pain is between the eyes and the nose is congested with nasal blockage, this suggests a sinus headache due to ethmoid sinusitis.

If the pain is in the cheek area and the teeth hurt, this indicates a problem either with the teeth or one of the maxillary sinuses. The same nerve, the inferior alveolar nerve (sometimes called the inferior dental nerve), serves both areas.

If the pain is vague but is associated with nasal congestion and there is evidence of some infection in the body, the headache may be due to a sphenoid sinus infection just behind the nose.

An ENT doctor can help make a definitive diagnosis. A telescopic exam of the sinus cavities with a telescope can reveal inflammation, blocked openings, mucus draining out of the sinuses, and anatomical problems like nasal polyps. A CT scan is a valuable aid in diagnosis.

Trevor came because he had sinus disease. No, he hadn't had pain or nasal blockage. He happened to have an MRI done two weeks ago when he fell off his bike. The doctor told him that he had sinus disease and that he should see an ENT specialist. I reviewed the MRI, which showed sinus changes. However, I explained to Trevor that the MRI picks up the slightest changes of mucus in the sinuses; it is simply too sensitive. Since I could find no evidence of disease on direct examination, I recommended that he ignore the MRI findings. (An MRI is not useful for diagnosing sinus disease. Any slight fluid is picked up on the film.)

Pain in the sinus area does not automatically mean that you have a sinus disorder. On the other hand, sinus and nasal passages can become inflamed leading to a headache. Headache is a key symptom of patients diagnosed with acute or chronic sinusitis. In addition to a headache, sinusitis patients often complain of pain and pressure around the eyes, across the cheeks and forehead; an achy feeling in the upper teeth; fever and chills; facial swelling; nasal stuffiness; and yellow or green discharge.

However, it is important to note that some cases of headache are related to chronic sinusitis without other upper respiratory symptoms. This suggests that an examination for sinusitis be considered when treatment for a migraine or other headache disorder is unsuccessful.

Rebecca, the mother of my patient, happened to mention that she had chronic fatigue syndrome, a severe tiredness that is not relieved by rest. Since her son Gustav had a chronic stubborn sinus problem, could her fatigue be due to sinus disease? It turns out that she did have an infected sinus, but with minimal nasal symptoms. The two had been passing the infection back and forth. Her fatigue was due to toxic byproducts caused by the sinus infection. An infected tooth, infected gums, a kidney infection, a sinus infection, and other localized areas of bacterial growth can affect the patient with symptoms of fatigue, fevers, and generalized aching, and requires very careful evaluation.

A WHOLE BODY APPROACH
TO ALLEVIATE SINUS HEADACHE PAIN

The key to relieving a sinus headache is to reduce the swelling and inflammation in the sinus cavities and to drain the mucus from them. There are a number of simple solutions that help prevent a sinus headache and alleviate its pain.

BREATHE MOIST AIR

Relief for a sinus headache can be achieved by humidifying the dry-air environment. A steam vaporizer or a cool-mist humidifier will help add moisture into the air. Inhaling steam from a basin of hot water (while covering the head and the bowl with a towel so the steam remains under the cloth) or from a long, steamy hot shower are alternatives; twice a day is preferred.

ALTERNATE HOT AND COLD COMPRESSES

Place a hot compress across your sinuses for three minutes and then replace it with a cold compress for 30 seconds. Repeat this procedure three times per treatment, two to six times a day, to reduce inflammation and pain.

USE PULSE-WAVE IRRIGATION

Ideally, nasal irrigation will remove bacteria and aid in healing. Avoid flowback devices like neti pots and squeeze bottles. The steady stream of solution from a pulse-wave irrigator is often best because it can open plugged sinuses and remove purulent material from the sinus cavities. When the pulse-wave irrigation restores the normal cilia activity, usually no further therapy is needed. For instructions, see page 54.

TAKE OVER-THE-COUNTER MEDICATIONS IF NEEDED

Some drugs are highly effective in reducing sinus headache pain. The primary ingredient in most over-the-counter pain relievers is aspirin, acetaminophen, ibuprofen, naproxen, or a combination of them. The best way to choose a pain reliever is by determining which of these ingredients works best for you.

USE DECONGESTANTS IF APPROPRIATE

Sinus pressure headaches caused by allergies are usually treated with decongestants and antihistamines. These medicines help reduce swelling inside the nose. In difficult cases, nasal steroid sprays may be recommended. Prescription antihistamine sprays such as Astepro work faster than corticosteroids and open the nasal and sinus passages. Benzedrex, an over-the-counter inhaler, works too. Benadryl, an over-the counter oral antihistamine opens nasal tissue and helps you sleep; therefore, 25 or 50 mg of Benadryl before sleep can be a big help.

Pseudoephedrine (Sudafed) is a popular over-the-counter oral decongestant that works over a period of hours. It is available in a short-acting (three-to-eight hour) 30-mg formula, and a longer-acting (twelve-hour) 120-mg formula. Some patients may get rapid heart with this product. Occasionally, someone may get a reverse reaction where they get sleepy with this, but that reaction is rare. Various combinations of Sudafed with antihistamines are available.

In my practice, for sinus pain and headache, I recommend a lozenge that contains a mixture of the anti-inflammatory fruit enzymes papain and bromelain. One lozenge taken four times a day helps reduce swelling in sinus cavities, which is often the factor in sinus headache pain. By reducing swelling due to inflammation, the closed sinus cavity can open up. Proteolytic enzymes (a group of enzymes that help digest protein as well as mucus) are best taken buccally (sucked on between the cheek and gums).

TRY HERBAL REMEDIES

Chinese herbalists use magnolia flower as a remedy for clogged sinus and nasal passages. In conjunction with other herbs, such as angelica, mint, and chrysanthemum, it is often recommended for upper respiratory tract infections and sinus headaches, although its effectiveness for these problems has not been scientifically confirmed.

OTHER HELPFUL HINTS TO CURE A HEADACHE

After reading this chapter you are well aware that there are many kinds of headaches. You can have a premenstrual headache one week, a migraine the next week, and a sinus headache the following week! Actually, there are simple headache solutions that will work irrespective of the actual etiology of the headache.

- Keep a headache diary. In it you record what might have been the trigger of your headache. You ate chocolate? You had a hangover? You slept late? Once you find that every time you ate grapes you got a headache, all you have to do is quit eating grapes.

- Relax your muscles. Any strain to muscles, especially the neck, can be a headache factor. Getting involved in a regular exercise program, having a massage, avoiding drafts and strains contribute to reducing all types of headaches.

- Practice measured breathing to lower the stress hormones and chemicals in your body. By preventing a buildup of unwanted stress chemicals, you will have fewer and less severe headaches.

- Breathe well. Good breathing may be as simple as clearing the nose and restoring cilia function. Once you do pulse-wave irrigation and the nose is open and clear, you will feel the difference.

- Get sufficient sleep each night: A daily routine of getting up and going to bed at the same time helps set the body's sleep clock, which promotes a deep sound sleep and makes for overall better health. Getting a good night's sleep is probably the most important headache prevention factor.

No matter what kind of headache you have, these last actions should be successful in reducing or clearing your symptoms. However, if none of these preventive measures or treatments is effective, a visit to an ENT specialist may be warranted. During the examination, a CT scan of the sinuses may be ordered to determine whether your headache is caused by a sinus infection. If no chronic sinusitis is found, treatment might then include allergy testing.

8

How to Clear Postnasal Drip and Thick Mucus

Postnasal drip is a very common complaint of my patients whether they have an allergy or sinusitis or a bad cold. With this condition, you are aware of a thick mucus or slime going down your throat. It is annoying, so you clear your throat or sometimes cough to clear it. If the thick liquid hangs in your larynx (voice box), it may interfere with breathing and with talking and singing. For singers and public speakers, postnasal drip can be a severe handicap. There is always a concern that it will affect your breath. Students are annoyed by the constant throat clearing when their teachers have postnasal drip.

Under normal conditions, your nose produces a quart of liquid every twenty-four hours. This fluid is an important first line of defense. It contains factors called immunoglobulins that act to take out bad bacteria. The harmful bacteria and other inhaled matter like dust and pollens are moved out of the nose within the mucus before they can enter the body. What mucus remains moves to the back of your throat where it moistens the lining of the throat and eventually slides down into the stomach. But with postnasal drip, the mucus moves too slowly and the bacteria have time to multiply and build up numbers that can enter your body. When the nasal cilia move too slowly, the normal mucus thickens and provides an environment in which bacteria can grow and thrive. The large number of bacteria can cause patients to feel constantly fatigued. The breath odor from this stagnant material depends on which bacteria flourish here.

In a congenital condition called cystic fibrosis, the mucus in the nose and lungs is so thick that the cilia can't move the bacteria out of the lungs or sinuses. As a result, serious bacterial infections occur frequently.

Currently, there are studies suggesting that in gastroesophageal reflux disease (GERD), the acid from the stomach reaches the nose and causes postnasal drip.

SYMPTOMS OF POSTNASAL DRIP

- Dry nasal passages
- Thick, sticky mucus in the throat
- Dry throat that can interfere with breathing, talking, and singing
- Feelings of a tickle or lump in the throat
- Coughing and frequent throat clearing
- Halitosis (bad breath)
- Hoarse, raspy voice

A WHOLE BODY APPROACH TO CLEAR POSTNASAL DRIP

The key to being clear of postnasal drip is keeping the mucus thin and the cilia moving. Try the following measures.

Thin Mucus Secretions

Increasing your intake of thinning agents such as lemon and lime will help break up thick mucus. You can do this easily by adding these to your drinking water. Try to drink eight 8-ounce glasses of water a day. Humming is effective because the vibration shakes up the mucus and breaks up the bonds that cause the thickness of the mucus.

Clear-ease is a lozenge I formulated that contains papain from papaya and bromelain from pineapple. When taken buccally, they significantly thin mucus. Clear-ease is particularly designed for speakers and singers to clear the thick mucus and reduce any laryngeal swelling. It is particularly effective for flyers and scuba divers who have difficulty clearing their ears due to heavy mucus or swelling. Because papain and bromelain are proteolytic enzymes, they break up the mucus bonds and thereby thin the mucus. These are taken four times a day. With thin mucus, the cilia can do their job.

Over-the counter mucous-thinning agents like guaifenesin (Mucinex) help thin secretions.

Increase Cilia Movement

To keep cilia moving, drink tea with lemon and honey throughout the day. The tea must be warm, not iced. (Remember, cold liquids slow the cilia.) Room temperature tea is okay but warm is best. Humming is effective. A low-toned "oooommmm" hummed for two minutes three times a day is effective too. Jumping rope and jumping jacks move the cilia as well. Putting your face near a soundboard (casing) of a vibrating source such as an organ or a piano works too.

My patient Jordan strongly objected to "oooommmm." He reported that humming the "Star Spangled Banner" was much more effective and was more patriotic.

Use Pulse-Wave Irrigation

Using pulse-wave irrigation for the nasal passages and sinuses is most effective because the pulse rate is ideal for breaking up the thick mucus as well as for stimulating the cilia. Think of the action like a vibration effect on water. Use the nasal irrigator twice a day. (For instructions, see page 54.) For patients with postnasal drip, I recommend adding two teaspoons of the sugar alcohol xylitol to the 16 ounces (500 ml) of saline solution in the irrigator basin. This will reduce any latent bacteria that may be responsible for the unwanted odor and taste. Note: xylitol doesn't actually kill the bacteria; instead, it reduces their ability to adhere to the tissue and most bacteria can't digest it. Two teaspoons of xylitol make a 1 percent solution. For some breath problems, it may be necessary to increase the concentration of the xylitol (four teaspoons make a 2 percent solution).

Some patients with postnasal drip also have biofilm. As you may recall, biofilm is an organized colony of certain bacteria. These bacteria are covered by a slime that makes it difficult for the xylitol or an antibiotic to penetrate. In such cases, add one teaspoon of Johnson's Baby Shampoo to the saline solution and irrigate the nasal passages twice a day. This shampoo is an inexpensive source of surfactin, a compound that loosens crusts and oily adhesions, which is why it is used for hair shampoo. I recommend the Johnson's product, as this is the item that has been used in research.

When I see a sinus patient who complains that the host of medications he or she has taken has failed to improve the postnasal drip, I look for biofilm. This is because the bacteria remain active under the biofilm blanket, despite that the patient is taking medications.

As I have repeated before, once the postnasal drainage condition is cleared, it is not necessary to continue pulse-wave irrigation. Once the nose is normal, it doesn't need to be more normal.

HOW TO PREVENT BAD BREATH

Under normal conditions, the mucus in your nose flows swiftly and removes stale material. If you drink enough fluids, your mouth stays fresh. Unfortunately, when people have sinus disease or postnasal drip, this is associated with slow cilia that cause the mucus to become stagnant. This allows various bacteria to multiply, leading to breath problems. Restoring good cilia movement with pulse-wave irrigation works here, but the process may also require removal of material that accumulates in crevices in the throat.

My Hydro-Pulse irrigation unit comes with two nasal tips and two throat tips, so you can attack the breath problem from the nose and the throat. For nasal irrigation, refer to the instructions on page 54. For throat irrigation, follow these directions:

1. Fill the irrigator basin with 16 ounces (500 ml) of warm water. You can use any solution–plain water, hydrogen peroxide, or a mouthwash such as Listerine. For example, add 1 tablespoon of an antiseptic solution such as Listerine mouthwash to the warm water.

2. Attach the throat irrigator attachment.

3. Place the throat irrigator on the right side of the tongue straight back. Aim the tip to spray the right side of the throat just behind the last tooth.

4. Bend way into the sink so you can see the drain.

5. Turn the machine on low. A stream of solution will go to the right side of the throat.

6. After using approximately one-half of the basin contents, turn off the machine and slide the tip to left side of the tongue. Aim the tip to left to strike just behind the last tooth and irrigate with the remainder of solution.

7. After use, rinse the irrigator thoroughly with clear water and dry it.

Another source of bad breath may be particles that have accumulated in the crevices of your tongue. For this reason, the throat irrigator tip has a tongue sweeper for removal of stale particles that cause breath problems too. With the tongue-sweeper part of the throat irrigator, you can sweep the tongue dry or irrigate with the solution at the same time. For my patients, the combination of throat irrigator, tongue sweeper, and nasal irrigator has been effective for typical breath problems.

Some other conditions in which the salivary glands reduce or quit making mucus or where there is less fluid intake include:

• Xerostomia: Dry mouth.

• Sialidinitis: Inflammation of the salivary glands (usually accompanied by dry mouth).

• Radiation therapy: The parotid gland on the back of the cheek and the submaxillary gland under the jaw (the glands that produce saliva) may show reduced saliva after radiation treatment (products such as Biotine Oral Rinse are of help).

- Fasting: A twenty-four hour fast without extra liquid.

- Low-carb diets: Certain chemicals are released in the breath as the body burns ketones (fats) for fuel.

- Certain medications: Antihistamines and diuretics (check for dryness with any new medication).

- Sleep: Saliva slows in sleep and allows bacteria to flourish.

Certain foods (of course, garlic being one) give odor and are another cause of bad breath. Chewing gum is recommended for the breath; gum is better than actual mints because it increases saliva flow.

Dental health is most important. If there is gum disease, this must be attended to, not only for the breath but to keep the teeth healthy as well. Drinking water will wash away stale bacteria. Lastly, don't forget the dental floss!

CLEAR UP YOUR ALLERGY, SINUSITIS, OR COLD

Previously you read that an allergy is usually a painless nasal congestion that can last a season, that chronic sinusitis is somewhat painful and is of shorter duration, and that a common cold lasts about a week with aching all over. Yet each can have postnasal drip as the primary complaint.

I regularly see patients who have tried everything for their postnasal drip without success. With a careful history and a food diary, some allergic cause usually shows up.

Francine was worried. When she visited her fiancé who lived in another city, she got heavy mucus that affected her throat and she worried about moving to this new city. Her food diary clearly showed that the take-out Chinese food her fiancé relished was the cause.

Taking antihistamines may dry the mucus excessively. A trial with one of the allergy prescription nasal sprays such as Astepro or Patanase is best so that the mucus membrane in the nose isn't dried too much.

THROAT COMPLAINTS THAT MAY MIMIC
OR BE CAUSED BY POSTNASAL DRIP

Many of the throat symptoms of burning, tickle, or swallowing difficulty can come from either postnasal drip or acid reflux and sometimes it is difficult to tell the exact cause. Although some mucus is naturally swallowed, when the mucus is thick and sticky it can feel as if it is congealing in the throat. But tight throat muscles can feel the same.

A Tickle in the Throat

Do you have a frequent, persistent dry cough, particularly at night? Viral infections, bronchitis, or GERD could be the cause. A tickle in the throat while singing may be caused by asthma and allergies but it also may be caused by irregular practice habits, laryngitis, secondhand smoke, or GERD.

Do you frequently clear your throat? This can be a symptom of asthma, but it can also be caused by postnasal drip, GERD, xerostomia, postnasal drip, and or voice disorders such as overuse and abuse of the vocal cords, nodes on the vocal cords, and more.

Is there a thick mucus rattling around on the vocal cords? Asthma, a virus, or sinusitis can be a cause.

If the remedies given in this chapter for postnasal drip don't clear the problem, having an ENT doctor look at your throat and vocal cords directly is best. The otolaryngologist will use a flexible laryngoscope that is passed through your nose (which is anesthetized) that will enable him or her to see if there is reflux (backup) from your stomach acid into the throat or if there is a condition of the vocal cords to be treated.

Common signs and symptoms of GERD include:

• Excessive thick phlegm, particularly in the morning

• Tired voice after regular use

• Heartburn

• Bad breath

- Bitter or sour taste in the mouth
- Chronic throat clearing and tickle in the throat
- Chronic, irritating cough
- A scratchy, sore throat, particularly in the morning
- Chronic hoarseness
- A lump in the throat
- Prolonged vocal warm-up, with low or husky voice quality
- Undependable voice—good one day, and hoarse and tired the next
- Trouble breathing or laryngospasm (closing off of the airway)
- Regurgitation of food and liquids
- Snoring

Recently, doctors have reported good results treating postnasal drip by prescribing proton-pump inhibitors such as omeprazole (Prilosec) for eight weeks. These medicines work by reducing the amount of stomach acid made by the stomach. The mechanism for this is not understood, but, if other methods fail, ask your doctor about such a trial. With the direct examination of the larynx with a laryngoscope, the doctor can accurately see if there is evidence of GERD and prescribe for it.

Fernando had been diagnosed with GERD and was being treated for it. But he continued to complain of a burning in his throat. When I looked at his larynx, the back of his vocal cords, which is adjacent to the esophagus, was distinctly red. It seems Fernando was taking his medication—a proton pump inhibitor—once at night (twice a day is the typical prescription). In addition, he hadn't raised the head of the bed in order to have gravity help to keep the stomach acid from coming into his throat. Also, he admitted to eating snack foods before bedtime. I explained the necessity of elevating the head of his bed four to six inches, stopping eating at least three hours before going to bed, and avoiding smoking and spicy foods. A month later Fernando was much better.

A Lump in the Throat

This is a common patient complaint. Patients often complain of a sensation of something stuck in the throat, a lump. It is not related to food intake, and it can come on at anytime and can last for hours. A patient may complain that nothing she has taken has helped. Other doctors have prescribed her alprazolam (Xanax) and similar relaxation medications. She had an upper gastrointestinal test called a barium swallow x-ray and this showed no foreign body.

This sensation is also a common complaint after removal of a foreign body. It is not unusual for patients to get a fish bone stuck in their throat and successfully removed on Friday night, and then to have them show up several days later insisting that the bone is still there!

Swallowing is a complex mechanism that involves major voluntary and involuntary throat muscles. Just as you get a "lump" when you flex your biceps, you can get a lump when any of the muscles that normally squeeze your food along bunch up or tighten or become spastic. Like any muscle contraction (such as the biceps), a lump can be felt.

To diagnose any of these throat complaints, the ENT first will take a careful history followed with a laryngoscopic evaluation to carefully examine the lower throat. Occasionally, the ENT can see a scratch or edema where a fishbone or object was removed. Usually, I can relieve the problem by palpating tightness in an associated cervical muscle. I also recommend the patient work on relaxing his or her neck and shoulder muscles by practicing measure breathing (breathing in for a count of four, then out for a count of six), while standing in front of a mirror to see the jaw and shoulders relax. Gentle throat exercises such as turning the neck and head from side to side are effective too. However, if GERD is present as a cause, this is diagnosed and treated. When you look at the larynx of someone with GERD, typically it is red, irritated, and swollen due to acid reflux damage.

Stress and nervousness are thought to trigger spasms that feel as if there is a lump in the throat. In my opinion, stress itself is not a cause but can aggravate the problem.

The timing of the symptoms may indicate a specific allergy as the cause; for example, the patient only gets this symptom after eating ice cream.

Cerebrospinal Fluid Fistula

Think of the top of the nose as the floor of the skull and brain. The brain is enclosed in a liquid medium called cerebrospinal fluid. Damage from some types of head injuries can cause an opening (fistula) from the brain envelope to the nose. This will result in a steady leakage of cerebrospinal fluid that can be mistaken for postnasal drip. When the drainage is clear, steady, and only on one side, that suggests a diagnosis of cerebrospinal fluid fistula; this can also occur without any injury or surgery.

A bone called the ethmoid bone serves as both the roof of the nose and the floor of the brain case. This bone is delicate and has thin walls. It is not difficult for an opening to be made through the ethmoid bone into the skull. This will also cause a steady leakage of fluid from the skull fluid system. This condition called a cerebrospinal leak is painless. The patient notes a steady liquid discharge that is not controlled by allergy pills or nasal sprays. His or her nasal passages are usually open and the airway is clear. As a rule, a doctor looking in the nose will not see the hole. But, by analyzing the fluid, a diagnosis can be made confirming whether it is cerebrospinal fluid. To help locate the opening, a radioactive dye can be inserted into the patient's spinal cord, which then travels to the nose and the discharge where it can be seen. Pledgets are placed in suspected areas of the nose and then measured to find the most likely area. When this fistula is caused at surgery, the patient complains of a headache that same day.

When a cerebrospinal leak is diagnosed after a head trauma or other injury, usually the doctor waits to see if the opening will close without treatment. During that wait, the patient must not blow his or her nose because that will force infected nasal material into the skull. Measures are used to reduce the fluid pressure as an aid to natural closure. If the fistula doesn't close, then a surgical closure is done.

9

HOW THE SINUSES AFFECT ASTHMA AND OTHER LUNG CONDITIONS

DID YOU KNOW THAT...?

- The speed of the cilia in the nose is usually the same speed of the cilia in airway passages.

- Over 70 percent of people with asthma have allergic rhinitis.

- Up to 40 percent of people with allergic rhinitis have asthma.

- More than 50 percent of people with asthma have sinusitis.

- Smoking is the primary cause of chronic obstructive pulmonary disease.

- Asthma symptoms are benefitted when a sinus infection or an allergy are cleared.

- Allergy to grass pollen is seen in people with allergic rhinitis and asthma.

Asthma, chronic obstructive pulmonary disease (COPD), cystic fibrosis, and other often life-threatening respiratory disorders are impacted by the health or ill health of your nose. After all, the nose normally filters airborne pollution particles and prevents them from entering the lungs. Air passes into the nose, down the throat, past the larynx, and then down the trachea (windpipe) where it divides into the two lungs. The bronchial passages get smaller and smaller, the smallest of which are called bronchioles, as the passages divide until the airway ends at tiny sack-like bubbles where oxygen and carbon dioxide are exchanged.

On inhalation the shoulders are raised to expand the lungs; the diaphragm descends to expand the lungs. People who practice singing and voice actually expand their lung capacity. Near the alveoli there are muscles that surround the bronchioles, which are supposed to relax on exhalation. In asthma these muscles are inflamed and narrowed.

How are the lungs and the sinuses related? In the embryo, the sinuses and the lungs develop from the same layer of cells. The nasal passages, sinuses, trachea, and bronchial passages have similar cilia and mucous-secreting cells. (Keep in mind the unified airway theory.) Whatever impairs the nasal cilia also impairs the cilia of the lungs. When the speed of the cilia in the nasal passages is measured, the speed of the cilia in the bronchial airways is often the same. Hospitalized patients with asthma, for example, will show nasal cilia that moves too slow and bronchial cilia that moves slowly too at about the same speed. Not surprisingly, challenges that affect the upper respiratory tract will likely affect the lower respiratory tract.

ASTHMA

The number of people with asthma continues to grow. One in twelve people (about 25 million, or 8 percent) of the U.S. population had asthma in 2009, compared with one in fourteen (about 20 million, or 7 percent) in 2001. An estimated 300 million people worldwide suffer from asthma, with 250,000 annual deaths attributed to the disease. It is estimated that the number of people with asthma will grow by more than 100 million by 2025. About 70 percent of asthmatics also have allergies.

Asthma is a disease that causes the airways of the lungs to swell and narrow, leading to shortness of breath, wheezing, a feeling of tightness in the chest, and coughing. It is the result of atopy, the inherited tendency to overreact to irritants in the environment. In your lungs, there are muscles that open the breathing passages and close them. Under normal conditions, these muscles relax the air passages as you exhale. During an asthma attack, the lining of the air passages swells and the muscles around the airways constrict the passages when you exhale. This tightness reduces the amount of air that can pass through the inflamed airway and produces the characteristic wheezing sound.

EARLY WARNING SIGNS OF ASTHMA

- Frequent cough, especially at night
- Losing your breath easily or shortness of breath
- Feeling very tired or weak when exercising
- Wheezing or coughing after exercise
- Feeling tired, easily upset, grouchy, or moody
- Decreases or changes in lung function as measured on a peak flow meter
- Signs of a cold or allergies (sneezing, runny nose, cough, nasal congestion, sore throat, and headache)
- Trouble sleeping

In an asthma attack, there is coughing that won't stop, wheezing when breathing both in and out, chest pain, difficulty in talking, and tightened neck and chest muscles. The neck area or space between the ribs may retract or sink in with each breath. The lips may be blue from lack of oxygen.

It is common to see patients with asthma who also have allergic rhinitis or sinusitis. In many people, these conditions coexist. Over 80 percent of patients with asthma manifest rhinitis symptoms and, furthermore, up to 40 percent of patients with rhinitis symptoms have asthma. Usually, a person will first develop allergic rhinitis or sinusitis or both, which then may lead to the development of asthma. If the patient has allergic rhinitis or chronic sinusitis, with a family history of asthma, doctors recommend allergy testing and desensitization. What is important is that anyone who starts to have asthma should have his or her sinus and nasal situation checked. Clearing a chronic sinus and/or allergy condition may prevent the advancement of asthma and worsening of the symptoms. If the sinus is infected, the body's reaction to that infection may be a significant factor in causing the asthma.

Other factors such as mouth breathing may be an important factor in making asthma worse. The purpose of nasal breathing is to filter, warm, and moisten the air before it reaches the lungs. With mouth breathing, the dry air entering the lungs can irritate the sensitive lung tissues and may precipitate an asthmatic attack. With mouth breathing, especially in a dusty workplace, the air to the lungs is not filtered and dust and bacteria enter easily. Breathing in cold air can also have the same effect in the airways. If the nose is blocked, inhaling cold air through the mouth might trigger the asthma. An asthma attack can also be triggered in atopic individuals by any number of irritants and allergens. Some of the more common asthma-provoking triggers are listed on page 142. Whatever the cause of the attack, it results in greater inflammation and narrowing in the airways, making exhaling more difficult.

MEASURING ASTHMA

A very important aid in the diagnosis and treatment of any respiratory problem such as asthma or COPD (discussed next) is a lung function test called spirometry. Spirometry is the main test doctors use to assess lung function. By measuring how much air comes in and out your lungs, the doctor can diagnose and treat you best. The test is done by breathing into a plastic tube—a spirometer—that is connected to a gadget that records the amount of air you can forcefully exhale. The volume of air you breathe out and the force with which it is exhaled is then measured for:

- Forced vital capacity (FVC): The total volume of air that can be forcibly exhaled indicates how large the lung is, how flexible it is, and how well the air passages open and close; FVC is reduced in asthma and COPD.

- Forced expiratory volume in one second (FEV1): The total volume of air that can be forcibly exhaled in one second; in asthma, the FEV1 is usually decreased and the FVC is normal; in COPD, both FEV1 and FVC are decreased.

A patient's FVC and the FEV1 are compared to normal values to evaluate lung capacity and function. There is a real advantage in making these measurements in order to gauge the severity of the airway function and the effectiveness of the therapy. With treatment, FVC and FEV1 measurements will be much improved because the lungs have opened up and there is much better air passage.

Other tests doctors may use for asthma include:

- Exercise-induced bronchoconstriction: This test measures the effect of exercise on the ability to pass air out quickly; it can occur in people with or without asthma.

- Methacholine challenge: A test for asthma that measures the effect of methacholine (a drug that constricts airways) on breathing; the more severe the asthma, the lower the dose that causes constriction. FEV1 is measured before and after the challenge.

UNDIAGNOSED ASTHMA

Asthma may be completely unrecognized and only manifest itself by seemingly minor annoyances such as a throat tickle, frequent throat clearing, a persistent dry cough, or a voice problem.

A tickle in the throat may be caused by asthma and allergies but also by GERD, laryngitis, or secondhand smoke.

Frequent throat clearing or a persistent dry cough can be a symptom of asthma, but can also be caused by GERD, xerostomia, postnasal drip, and voice disorders involving overuse/abuse and nodules (small growths that develop on the vocal cords).

If there is a thick mucus rattling around on the vocal folds, asthma, a virus, or sinusitis can be a cause.

Note: A tight chest, wheezing, and shortness of breath with moderate exertion is a frequent sign of undiagnosed asthma. Go to the doctor immediately. Shortness of breath may only show by pausing in the middle of a sentence to take a breath. Non-asthmatics finish several sentences before taking a breath.

A WHOLE BODY APPROACH TO ASTHMA RELIEF

Asthma requires careful diagnosis and treatment and is not a condition that patients should self-treat. Yes, you still need to do your asthma exercises and take your preventive medications, but the WBA can reduce your asthma symptoms and can make a big difference between health and treatment failure.

TAKE MEDICATIONS IF NEEDED

There are two kinds of medicines for treating asthma: short-acting medicines for use during attacks and long-acting medicines to help control or prevent attacks.

Short-acting medications for quick relief of symptoms during an asthma attack include albuterol (Proventil), pirbuterol (Maxair), and metaproterenol (Alupent). These medicines are generally available as inhaled bronchodilators. They are referred to as *beta2-adrenergic agonists,* or beta2-agonists, because they act on the beta2-adrenergic receptor. This action causes the smooth muscles that might narrow the bronchial airways on exhalation to relax and stops the asthma symptoms. These are inhaled through the mouth so that they go directly to the lungs. Important: On inhaling these medications, take a deep inhalation, then hold for at least ten seconds to get full absorption of the medication.

Long-acting asthma medications such as salmeterol (Serevent Discus) and formoterol (Symbicort) are taken on a regular basis to prevent and control potential asthma attacks. These long-acting beta2-agonists do not relax the airways but instead help reduce inflammation over time. Various combinations of these long- and short-acting drugs are also available. For example, the inhaler Advair Diskus comes as a powder containing a combination of fluticasone propionate and salmeterol. Fluticasone is a short-acting steroid that reduces bronchial inflammation and salmeterol is a long-acting beta2-agonist that relaxes bronchial smooth muscles with little effect on the heart rate. For various patients, this may work well.

Whichever beta-agonist is used, the side effects may include rapid heart rate, tremor, sweats, and agitation. Unusual side effects include pulmonary edema, heart attack, and arrhythmia (irregular heart rhythm). If you are taking these medications, keep a list of them in your wallet in the same pocket as your driver's license—this simple act could save your life.

Leukotriene inhibitors include montelukast (Singulair), zafirlukast (Accolate), and zileuton (Zyflo). Leukotrienes are immune system compounds that, in excess, produce damaging chemicals that cause inflammation and spasms in the airways of people with asthma. Leukotriene inhibitors block the binding of leukotriene D4 to its receptor. This blockage reduces allergic and asthma symptoms. In some patients taking 10 mg of Singulair daily can significantly reduce allergy and asthma symptoms.

Cromylyn (Intal) is a *mast cell stabilizer.* It has both anti-inflammatory and antihistamine properties. When used as an over-the-counter nasal spray, called NasalCrom, it may avoid allergy symptoms. It is used two to four weeks before the allergy season, three to four times a day. Preventing the mast cells from releasing histamine may prevent any allergy symptoms during the pollen season. Using NasalCrom has few side effects.

Ipratropium (Atrovent) is an *anticholinergic drug* that is given by nasal spray. It works by decreasing nasal secretions and is primarily used in non-allergic rhinitis. Atrovent HFA is used as an inhaler to treat chronic bronchospasms. It is an anticholinergic that inhibits vagus nerve reflexes, causing the muscles surrounding the airways to relax and enlarge.

The newest treatment for asthma is omalizumab (Xolair), a *monoclonal anti-IgE antibody,* a genetically developed drug designed to attack very specific targets. Xolair is given by injection every two to four weeks. It neutralizes circulating IgE and prevents it from triggering the inflammatory events that lead to an asthma attack. Xolair is indicated in some forms of urticaria (skin allergy).

The WBA is most important in asthma. Understanding what medications are for, following directions, reducing anxiety, and eating a proper diet all make the difference between health and treatment failure. Every study shows that trips to the emergency room are a result of the patient not following instructions, misplacing the inhaler or not using it correctly or worse. When a visiting nurse is sent to the home to make sure that the treatment program is being followed, then death rates drop and so do trips to the emergency room. In asthma and other lung conditions, clearing the sinuses of any disease is essential. If the non-surgical means are insufficient, then good results can be expected with the surgical therapies of today.

DO LUNG-STRENGTHENING EXERCISES

Breathing exercises are often part of an asthmatic's treatment as they help strengthen the lungs and increase their capacity. You need to practice measured breathing on page 50. The slow relaxed breathing reduces inflammation and trains you to avoid rapid anxiety breathing. For asthma, do the breathing exercises for five minutes four times a day.

Measured breathing is only one form of exercise. Your doctor or physical therapist may recommend a program especially for you. For children, the parent should demonstrate the asthma exercise so the child can follow the parent.

IDENTIFY ASTHMA TRIGGERS

You need to learn what triggers your asthma and then reduce your exposure to them. Your triggers are not the same as your brother's. The most common asthma-provoking triggers to look for are:

- Air pollution
- Cold moist air
- Extreme dryness
- Foods and food additives (learn yours)
- GERD (also known as heartburn)
- Hormonal fluctuations that worsen before menstruation

- High humidity

- Inadequate hydration

- Medications such as angiotensin-converting enzyme inhibitors, aspirin and aspirin-related products, and beta-blockers that block adrenaline effects

- Moist air with fungal spores

- Odors (paint fumes, formaldehyde, solvents, etc.)

- Pollen allergy (trees, grasses, weeds)

- Sinusitis

- Strenuous physical activity

- Stress

- Tobacco smoke

- Viral and chest infections

SAMTER'S TRIAD

Samter's triad is a severe form of asthma that results from a combination of nasal polyps, treatment-resistant asthma, and sensitivity to aspirin and non-steroidal anti-inflammatories (NSAIDS). People with this condition develop a rash or asthmatic reaction, which can be life threatening, when they take aspirin and aspirin-related medications. The condition usually occurs in those past age thirty who have a history of frequent chest infections and nasal polyps. People with Samter's triad must avoid aspirin and non-steroidal anti-inflammatory products.

RESOLVE AN ALLERGY AND/OR SINUS CONDITION

Anyone who starts to have asthma symptoms should have his or her sinus situation checked. Clearing a chronic sinus condition may prevent the advancement of asthma; the same applies to allergy. Because allergic rhinitis and sinusitis often go hand in hand with asthma, once asthma starts to develop, it may be best to start pulse-wave irrigation (for instructions, see page 54). Improving nasal cilia function helps respiratory function as well. If the sinuses are infected, the body's reaction to that infection may be a significant factor in causing the asthma; therefore, prevention and treatment of asthma can be accomplished by eliminating the sinus infection. (For a review of the WBA for resolving allergies and sinusitis, see Chapters 3 and 5, respectively.)

CULTIVATE A HAPPY AFFECT

There is little question that stress can be a trigger for asthma. To put it bluntly, there is nothing funny about having asthma. Yet, the science of psychoneuroimmunology has shown that smiling can reduce your symptoms. Studies of smiling have demonstrated that smiling really does activate the brain to release good chemicals that raise your immune factors, whereas feeling depressed reduces your immune factors, making you more liable to stay sick. There's no question that maintaining a happy smiling face while having an asthmatic attack will make a lot of people wonder about your mental state. But maybe with humor you won't get that attack. How can you feel happy when you are struggling to breathe properly?

The key is to cultivate a happy affect. Of course, you won't feel funny and happy all the time. But if you laugh and feel joy 90 percent of the time, you will build up the good chemicals to keep you healthy. If Alphonso could do it, so can anyone. He was disabled with a serious injury. He had been on the floor level at the elevated loading dock. A truck went to unload and crushed him against the wall, breaking nearly every rib. Essentially, he was unable to breathe for several minutes until the truck withdrew. Every time he saw his therapists he had funny stories to tell them. I am sure he got better faster. (See below on how to develop a humor habit.)

It is important to understand that stress is not a cause of asthma; it can act as a trigger to people with atopy and allergy.

HOW TO DEVELOP A HUMOR HABIT

You can develop a humor habit. Here are some exercises from my book *Stressed? Anxiety? Your Cure is in the Mirror:*

- Practice memorizing short shopping lists using humor.

- Rent comedies and write down funny scenes to describe them to others.

- Find comedy websites and blogs and record the best ones to tell your friends.

- Borrow humor DVDs, books, and tapes from your local library.

- Pretend you are a TV writer and once a week write a funny TV show.

- If you see a funny episode on TV, carry it in your mind to tell your friend next evening. Instead of stressful or anxious thoughts, your thoughts will dwell on laughter throughout the day.

- Find someone or a group to swap jokes with.

- Pretend you are an actor who is playing a happy role. Record a comedy show and pretend you are playing the comic role. When you do this you change your body chemistry. Blood samples taken when a fine actor plays a sad, sad role one week, and taken again the next week when he plays a happy, happy role actually show a chemical difference. Playing ("pretending") the happy role is healthier.

DON'T FORGET THE WARM TEA

Since we know that warm green or black tea (with or without caffeine) stimulates nasal cilia, then it is also beneficial for asthmatics, especially when there are symptoms of wheezing and shortness of breath. The same benefit of L-theanine in tea also benefits the cilia of the lungs.

IF YOUR SYMPTOMS ARE NOT IMPROVING, CONSIDER THESE FACTORS

Asthma may be improved by attention to these factors:

1. Are you following instructions properly? As simple a factor as not using the inhaler correctly can aggravate asthma. Of all the factors affecting asthma, the number one cause of poor outcome is failure to follow medication instructions properly. Studies show that when patients are given extra counseling and are tested to see if they are

using their inhalers correctly, their asthma improves. Of all the medical conditions discussed in this book, applying medication enhancement (see page 45) to asthma is the most significant.

2. Is sinusitis a factor in treatment failure? When sinus disease is cleared, asthmatics generally improve.

3. Is GERD a factor in treatment failure? Your stomach secretes acid for food digestion. There is a sphincter muscle that pinches off the opening between the esophagus tube above and the stomach below. This sphincter may be ineffective and may allow stomach acid to flow back into the throat and find its way into the lungs. Because the acid is highly irritating, it can cause asthmatic symptoms. Typically, GERD occurs in a person who eats a heavy meal late at night and then goes to bed, lying flat. The full stomach overcomes the sphincter action and the acid is pushed up the esophagus into the throat, and then falls into the lungs. If GERD is left untreated, it can eventually damage the lining of the throat, airways, and lungs, making breathing difficult and often causing a persistent cough. Smoking weakens the sphincter that shuts off the stomach acid, as does alcohol.

To prevent GERD, you should avoid eating after eight o'clock and raise the head of your bed as much as is comfortable; the higher your back is, the more benefit from gravity and the harder it is for the acid to go upward. Lying on your left side is much better than lying flat or on your right side.

CHRONIC OBSTRUCTIVE PULMONARY DISEASE

There are two main types of COPD: chronic bronchitis, which involves a long-term cough, and emphysema, which involves progressive damage to the lungs. People with COPD may have one form or both. Either may compromise lung function. COPD is often found in heavy smokers and in people who are chronically exposed to heavy dust and chest irritants. COPD is caused by noxious particles or gas, most commonly from tobacco smoking, which triggers an abnormal inflammatory response in the lung. COPD is the third leading cause of death in the United States.

Symptoms of COPD are chronic cough, coughing up phlegm, and shortness of breath (dyspnea). There is limited airflow: the FEV1 (the amount of air expired in one minute) is reduced, as is the total amount of expired air. People with COPD commonly describe this as: "My breathing requires effort," "I feel out of breath," or "I can't get enough air in." People with COPD typically first notice the dyspnea during vigorous exercise when the demands on the lungs are greatest. Over the years, dyspnea tends to get gradually worse so that it can occur during milder, everyday activities such as housework. In the advanced stages of COPD, dyspnea can become so bad that it occurs during rest and is constantly present.

Normally, as you inhale tiny air sacs in the lungs called alveoli expand as air comes in and contract as air exits. Due to inflammation, excess mucus, and smoke irritation, the expansion of the alveoli becomes permanent. The remaining expanded alveoli reduce the effectiveness of oxygen absorption by the lungs. The expansion of the lungs also causes the chest to deform and become rounded; people with COPD often develop a barrel chest.

Other symptoms of COPD are sputum or mucous production, wheezing, chest tightness, and tiredness.

SIGNS OF COPD

- Shortness of breath
- Breathing through pursed lips
- Rapid breathing (tachypnea)
- Wheezing sounds or crackles in the lungs heard through a stethoscope
- Longer time needed to breathe out than to breathe in
- Enlargement of the chest, particularly the front-to-back distance, a barrel chest
- Active use of muscles in the neck to help with breathing

Changes in the airways reduce the rate at which air can flow to and from the alveoli and limits the effectiveness of the lungs. In COPD, the greatest reduction in airflow occurs when breathing out (during expiration), because the pressure in the chest tends to compress rather than expand the airways. In theory, airflow could be increased by breathing more forcefully, increasing the pressure in the chest during expiration. In COPD, there is often a limit to how much this can actually increase airflow, a situation known as expiratory flow limitation.

If the rate of airflow is too low, a person with COPD may not be able to completely finish breathing out (expiration) before he or she needs to take another breath. This is particularly common during exercise, when breathing has to be faster. A little of the air of the previous breath remains within the lungs when the next breath is started, resulting in an increase in the volume of air in the lungs, a process called dynamic hyperinflation.

By far, the most common cause of COPD is tobacco smoking; the more a person smokes, the more likely that person will develop COPD—approximately 80 percent of COPD deaths are caused by smoking. Besides smoking, certain occupational exposures increase the risk for COPD. Intense and prolonged exposure to workplace dusts found in coal mining, gold mining, and the cotton textile industry, and to chemicals such as cadmium, isocyanates, and fumes from welding have been implicated in the development of airflow obstruction, even in nonsmokers. Wood workers get COPD both from wood and the solvents and paints they use. Workers who smoke and are exposed to these particles and gases are even more likely to develop COPD. Intense silica dust exposure causes silicosis, a restrictive lung disease distinct from COPD; however, less intense silica dust exposures have been linked to a COPD-like condition. The effect of occupational pollutants on the lungs appears to be substantially less important than the effect of cigarette smoking.

Air pollution also increases a person's risk for COPD. In all countries, the incidence of COPD is higher in large cities than in urban areas. Wherever there are sulfur dioxide products, these can combine with other products and end up as a form of sulfuric acid, a strong, corrosive chemical that causes severe burns and tissue damage! In developing countries, indoor pollution from cooking fire smoke is a common cause of COPD, particularly in women. Even such a simple thing as a poorly vented fireplace can be a factor, including wood burning stoves. Gas stoves? Many doctors insist that their patients switch to electric stoves. Cooking should be done with a working hood that is well ventilated.

In COPD there is poor air exchange; often air is trapped so that fresh air is blocked by old air. There can be a significant build up of carbon dioxide (CO_2) with low oxygen levels.

Diagnosing COPD

People over forty who complain of shortness of breath, have a chronic cough and heavy sputum production, with a smoking history, are possible COPD patients. The standard test for COPD is spirometry, the lung function test discussed earlier in the chapter. The test involves exhaling as hard as possible into a spirometer that tests your lung capacity.

A WHOLE BODY APPROACH TO COPING WITH COPD

COPD cannot be cured. Yet there are many things you can do to relieve symptoms of the disease and to keep it from getting worse. There are medications you can take but by far the best way to slow down damage to your lungs is to quit smoking. There are excellent COPD support groups (see Resources' section) and many hospitals offer exercise programs that can be of benefit in increasing the airway response.

TAKE MEDICATIONS FOR COPD IF NEEDED

Anticholinergic drugs and corticosteroids are commonly used to help control symptoms of COPD.

Anticholinergic medications cause the smooth muscles in the bronchial airways to relax by blocking stimulation from cholinergic nerves. Ipratropium (Atrovent) provides short-acting rapid relief of COPD symptoms. Tiotropium (Spiriva) is a long-acting anticholinergic whose regular use is associated with improvements in airflow, exercise capacity, and quality of life. Both medications are generally inhaled.

Corticosteroids are used in tablet or inhaled form to treat and prevent acute exacerbations of COPD. Inhaled corticosteroids have not been shown to be of benefit for people with mild COPD; however, they have been shown to decrease acute exacerbations in those with either moderate or severe COPD. Their use has no effect on overall one-year mortality and is associated with increased rates of pneumonia.

Newer medications include *phosphodiesterase inhibitors.* One such phosphodiesterase inhibitor is theophylline (Theolair), a bronchodilator that in high doses can reduce symptoms for some people who have COPD. Phosphodiesterase is an enzyme that causes inflammation in the airways and that is overproduced in COPD. More often, side effects such as nausea and stimulation of the heart limit its use. Two phosphodiesterase-4 antagonists, roflumilast (Daxas) and cilomilast (Ariflo), have completed Phase 2 (mid-stage) clinical trials and their use for COPD is pending approval. Also, tumor necrosis factor (TNF) antagonists such as infliximab (Remicade) reduce inflammation. There are excellent COPD support groups (see Resources' section). Many hospitals offer exercise programs that can be of benefit in increasing the airway response. They also offer support groups for smoking cessation.

QUIT SMOKING

Many people find it very difficult to quit smoking. Smoking is habit forming because it releases dopamine, a pleasure-releasing chemical in the brain; thus, it acts as a stress reducer. You smoke for relaxation.

Smoking cessation drugs include nicotine patches (NicoDerm), which deliver nicotine through the skin; bupropion (Zyban), a type of antidepressant used for smoking cessation; and varenicline (Chantix), a newer drug that may work better than Zyban. Whichever method is used, belief in the method and the patient taking charge of the method is needed.

Why not try the WBA method instead? The reason it works is because it addresses the cause for your smoking: tension and stress. This method reduces both. You smoke for energy. By reducing your stress, you increase your energy. When you use all five of your senses plus joy, the habit is changed to seeking more of that non-smoking joy.

Is there proof that this works? In the latest drug study of success in smoking cessation, 44 percent of the participants had success in quitting smoking long term using the drug. But 25 percent quit and stayed quit with the placebo! Therefore, if you follow this action plan, you will be taking charge of your health and you will have all the tools needed to quit. For instructions, see below.

George used a blank pad to draw an outline of the lungs. Every day he drew a picture of lungs and colored them brown and black. Each day he reduced or stopped smoking, he drew the lungs as less brown and more pink.

Both of Fred's parents had smoker's cough and were anxious that Fred, at seventeen, quit smoking. Finally, when Fred asked for help in getting a car, his dad offered help if he didn't smoke for six months. This worked and Fred never went back to smoking.

Rosalyn knew as much about the bad effects of smoking as any doctor, yet she continued to smoke. When her hair stylist commented that smoking ages the skin and causes you to look older, she quit smoking.

To repeat: you smoke for relaxation. These ten actions will give you relaxation. You smoke because of stress. These actions relieve stress.

HOW TO STOP SMOKING FROM *STRESSED? ANXIETY? YOUR CURE IS IN THE MIRROR*

Do these ten actions daily in order to change your brain circuitry. If all you do is read this information without actually doing the actions, it's the same as learning to play tennis by reading a book. Only by daily repetition will your circuits be reprogrammed. Best of all, you can't get an allergic reaction by doing this daily.

1. Breathe in to a count of four. Do this for a minute. By counting to four with each inhalation you regulate the breathing. Think of clean air coming in to replace the built-up cigarette tar.

2. For one minute concentrate on breathing out for a count of six. Exhalation is a

relaxation mode, so the longer the exhalation, the more you are in a relaxed state. Imagine the tar and tobacco stains leaving your larynx and lungs. Imagine some toilet paper catching the exhaled air and the brown gunk ending up on it. Taste the tar that is coming up.

3. For one minute, breathe in to a count of four and out for a count of six. As you exhale, let the exhalation be a signal to your body to relax. As you exhale, visualize the dirty yellow air in your smoker's lungs leaving your body, to leave it healthier.

4. Now use the mirror as a biofeedback device. Above your eyes is the frontalis muscle (the one that contracts when you worry), so make sure that it is relaxed. First, contract or squeeze your frontalis muscle area as with worry, and then relax it. See that by not smoking your skin gets a nicer color and fewer wrinkles. As you reduce your smoking, see the skin becoming healthier. Continue breathing in for a count of four and out for a count of six. See clean air and fields of green grass.

5. Next see and feel your jaw relax in the mirror. The jaw is one of the main muscles of anxiety and stress. Our ancestors needed to use the mouth for fighting, and thousands of people have TMJ, a condition characterized by pain in the jaw joint and pain on yawning. (Note: Don't open your mouth. Relax the muscles of your jaw so that it falls open by gravity—like when your dad falls asleep while watching TV.) Continue the measured breathing. By this time you should be nicely relaxed. Start giving yourself affirmations: "I will reduce my smoking," "I will only take two puffs and put the cigarette out," "I will not smoke a cigarette until after supper." As long as some sort of input comes in, that is desirable. The affirmations must be repeated in synchrony to the exhaled breathing and repeated very often. You smoke to hold something in your mouth to sooth the jaws or to give something for your jaws to do. Once you properly relax your jaw, you won't need the cigarettes for this anymore.

6. See and feel the shoulders relax in the mirror. This is best done looking to the mirror until it is learned, and then it can be done without the mirror. Continue with measured breathing, except on the exhalation let that be a signal to relax the shoulders. Visualize clean air coming in and dirty air going out. (As you exhale, you really are releasing cigarette elements.) Visualize a clean, fresh pink lung as you see the shoulders relax. Get some indigo crayons and color some objects you

keep in your purse. Put paint samples of indigo in your purse or wallet to remind you of this shoulder relaxation, with emphasis on breathing out the bad tar and breathing in clean air. When you do this, you relax; picture the lungs as a sponge that is squeezing out brown gunk.

7. Recall when you didn't smoke. Use your five senses plus joy. Recall a good athletic time or winning a race using all five senses. Spending time this way will reproduce the good chemistry that you are missing due to your smoking. Notice how different your skin looks.

8. Relax from the toes up. This is the progressive relaxation technique first advocated by Dr. Edmund Jacobson, a specialist in tension control, fifty years ago. It is an excellent way to get a full-body relaxation. Initially, you should contract or squeeze the muscle, and then relax it. Later you can go right to relaxation. Start with the toes and move up to the pelvis, abdomen, and chest, then to the fingers, forearms, arms, and shoulders, and then to the neck, jaw, face, and forehead. As you are relaxing, imagine the dirty smoke-stained tissue being exhaled.

9. Raise one finger. Do three measured breaths. On the third breath, let your finger drop and touch the desk or your body. When it touches, let that be your signal to relax. It is very important to spend time on this. This is a conditioned reflex that you can use while driving or before any stressful situation. Once learned, it can significantly improve your efficiency as well as your health. I teach this to scuba divers and they use far less air on diving. For the smoker, this is the signal you should use when the urge for a cigarette comes on. Also, if you hold a cigarette or a pack of cigarettes, the fingers will remind you of this signal. When you drop the finger, you crush an unlit cigarette. Or you can visualize a cartoon of Mr. Cigarette and crush him when you drop the finger. Or you can actually crush a cigarette or a picture of one for reinforcement.

10. Go to a healing place. We talk about healing places and the fact that they work. Science has demonstrated that many of the same benefits that can be achieved by visualization as long as you use all five senses. Imagine being on a beautiful sailboat. The air is fresh and clean. See the waves, hear the wind in the sails, smell the ocean air, taste the salty water in your mouth, and feel the railing of the boat. You feel relaxed here. You appreciate that the air can now get all the way into your lungs because the tobacco tar is no longer impeding the transfer of oxygen

to your body. Imagine landing at a dock and going to the bubbling pool that everyone says has healing powers. You enter the pool, it is warm and relaxing, and you really do feel good. The water has a mineral-like smell. You taste it, and it is somewhat bitter but has a hint of lemon. After a while, you are fully relaxed and exit the pool, whereupon you are wrapped in a giant terry cloth towel and fall soundly asleep on a couch. When you awake, you feel refreshed and vibrant. Every other day alternate this visualization with the following one: Recall all the people you know who have coughed because of smoking. Visualize their coughing and bringing up phlegm. Recall some of the anti-smoking advertisements of the muscular man with COPD who can't even blow out a candle because of his smoking. Every hour, on the hour, think of a green forest or field.

To repeat, many people find it difficult to stop smoking. If you repeat these ten actions daily you will build up new tracks in your body that will correct your habit and make for overall health.

AND DON'T FORGET . . .

I have had my COPD patients use humming in order to break up the thick phlegm and reduce the cough. Honey may ease the constant cough. Papain and bromelain proteolytic enzymes might thin the mucus and inflammation. Warm green tea may help reduce the sputum by stimulating cilia.

10

HOW TO TREAT THROAT AND VOICE PROBLEMS

HERE ARE TEN VOICE HELPERS:

- If your voice is hoarse, rest it.
- Do not gargle.
- Don't yell and scream when your team is winning.
- Don't yell and scream when your team is losing.
- Inhale steam through your mouth with your tongue out.
- Increase your intake of lemon and lime drinks.
- Use menthol cough drops.
- Never use force against a "weak" voice.
- Good posture is a must.
- Use mirror biofeedback to relax throat muscles.

Muscle tension is a major cause of voice problems. Try this: look straight ahead and say out loud, "When I wake up in the morning I feel rested and refreshed." Now say this with your head turned sharply to the right; then repeat the phrase with your head turned to the left. The difference in your voice comes from the tension of the throat muscles.

THROAT MUSCLES AND VOCAL CORDS

Your head is balanced with an equal pull on the front and back cervical muscles. But when you are tense, both sets of muscles tighten. Your head remains balanced but the muscles are tense and this affects the voice muscles. Singing teachers work to keep those throat muscles relaxed so that the vocal cords are not impeded or strained.

Look at opera singers. Notice how they relax their head before starting a long solo such as an aria. Notice the top boxers. Some of them look half asleep! They have learned to relax before throwing a punch so that the front muscles are thrusting 100 percent and are not impeded by the backward muscles being tight.

Vocal technique—speaking and singing—is a learned response. How we use our voices is a learned technique. The technique becomes automatic, and we are seldom consciously aware of how we use our voices. Sometimes your voice is hoarse one day and seems almost normal the next (day-to-day variability), so you tend to ignore a problem, unless you earn your living with your voice.

SIGNS OF VOICE AND THROAT PROBLEMS

(courtesy of voice specialist Rosalie Loeding)

- Coughing, throat tickle, and throat clearing
- Heavy breathing and wheezing
- Poor posture
- Indigestion
- Bloating
- Acid taste in mouth (acid reflux)
- Loss of voice
- Excessive tension or muscle tightness
- Excess voice fatigue

It helps to think of the vocal cords as two hands clapping. If you clap gently and evenly, then the hands stay healthy. If you clap very strongly for a long time, then the skin gets raw and you get calluses and uneven areas. Now, visualize your shoulders becoming very tight. Try and clap, and you'll see that you can't clap as well. And, if you have, say, a bad shoulder or back, you'll have even more difficulty clapping.

The same applies to your vocal cords. After shouting all afternoon at the ball game, the surfaces of the vocal cords will be swollen. If your neck is held tightly, that pulls on the larynx and affects how the vocal cords come together (the tighter the neck, the more strained the voice). Singing teachers tell their pupils to practice in front of a mirror. With the mirror, they can see if their face, shoulders, and jaw are relaxed. Note: Originally a performer in Australia, Frederick Matthias Alexander (1869–1955), cured his own hoarseness by using mirrors to see if his muscles were relaxed. This developed into a method of mind-muscle therapy called the Alexander Technique that is still taught today.

DIAGNOSING THROAT AND VOICE PROBLEMS

Problems of the voice are usually referred to an ENT specialist by the voice teacher.

HOARSENESS

Do you have a frequent, persistent dry cough, particularly at night? Viral infections, bronchitis, or GERD could be the cause. A tickle in the throat that occurs during singing may be caused by irregular practice habits, GERD, laryngitis, or secondhand smoke, but also by asthma and allergies. It's most important to check your nose for drainage and congestion. Drainage from postnasal drip can accumulate on the vocal cords and affect the voice. Allergy seldom affects the larynx directly; however, drainage from nasal allergy or chronic sinusitis can accumulate on the vocal cords. If the mucus is thick, it may lodge directly on the vocal cords and be difficult to clear.

Do you frequently clear your throat? This can be a symptom of asthma but it can also be caused by GERD, xerostomia, postnasal drip, and voice disorders such as overuse and abuse of the vocal cords, nodules, or some other throat condition.

Is there a thick mucus rattling around on the vocal cords? Asthma, a virus, or sinusitis can be a cause. Make sure you are drinking enough liquids. Also, consider taking Clear-ease, a lozenge I formulated that contains the proteolytic enzymes papain and bromelain. These enzymes reduce swelling and thin the mucus by breaking up the mucus bonds. Since the enzymes are inactivated by stomach acid, it is best to melt the lozenges in the buccal (cheek) pouch. Take one lozenge four times a day. Many of my patients who are performers use Clear-ease at the slightest onset of a voice change.

A food allergy also can be the cause of a tickle in throat and mucus accumulation. Try using a food diary to track down the suspected food (for directions, see page 111). If either of these symptoms is worse when you drink red wine or certain foods, try omitting the food or drink for two weeks. But be sure to add the suspected trigger back in gradually to see if the symptoms come back so that you have a real answer. For example, if one suspect food is bread, you need to look at the related-wheat products that need to be avoided.

Singers, in particular, have difficulty with GERD. With GERD, there is increased intra-abdominal pressure associated with voice training. This naturally pushes against the sphincter, the muscle that normally separates the stomach from the esophagus. That extra pressure that is used when singers and actors project the voice may weaken that muscle. When the sphincter or valve is weak, it is easy for stomach acid to go out of the stomach and up the esophagus. Then the acid can reach the larynx or even the nose.

Another problem is that performers may not eat before the evening performance, and they come home late, eat a heavy meal, and go to bed. That flat position with an active stomach acid is a sure way to weaken the sphincter. See more on acid reflux and GERD in Chapter 8.

HEAVY BREATHING

A tight chest, wheezing, and shortness of breath with moderate exertion should send up a red flag. Go to the doctor immediately. Do you feel that you need a breath before completion of a relatively short phrase? Poor posture inhibits relaxed deep breathing. Try the following to experience the effect of poor posture on breathing:

- Pull your shoulders up and forward, and try to take a deep breath.

- Slump with your arms forward, cave the ribcage in, and try to take a deep breath.

Both of these behaviors restrict the expansion of the ribcage.

The head and chin raised or jutting forward may be an asthmatic's compensation for an inability to take a deep, relaxed breath. This produces tension of the extrinsic neck muscles and the stretched, tense neck muscles make it impossible for the vocal folds to work properly. The sound is strained. (Of course, it can be caused by straining to reach a high note.)

People who have had voice or singing lessons have expanded lung capacity. If they then develop a voice problem from asthma, their lung studies may show good airway, yet their voice is affected and they need therapy. When the head, neck, and spine are correctly aligned, breathing and muscle tension problems resolve. Fortunately, heavy breathing due to asthma responds to medication. If it is treated early, the problem can be fully relieved. But if it is ignored and left untreated, changes in the airways and the microscopic area of the lung may occur that are irreversible.

EXCESSIVE MUSCLE TENSION

Tension in the chest wall is often the result of constriction of airways and can cause tight vocal muscles, leading to early fatigue.

Excessive tension in the muscles of the face, neck, and particularly in the jaw, is a common cause of voice disability.

Tension of the extrinsic and intrinsic neck muscles (located above and below the voice box) can also be caused by poor vocal technique and poor posture, as well as by emotional stress and TMJ.

For excessive tension in any of these muscles, the biofeedback exercises described on pages 116–117 for TMJ work for most people.

SIGNS OF EXCESS MUSCLE TENSION

- Fatigue after normal activities without sufficient cause.

- A wrinkled forehead, indicating tension.

- Appearance of nervousness, restlessness, or irritability (the "short-fuse syndrome") can be caused by tension.

- Pain while speaking or singing is usually the result of vocal abuse and bad technique.

- Other causes of excess muscle tension include GERD, infection, arthritis of the arytenoids joints (joints in the larynx), and poor singing technique.

A WHOLE BODY APPROACH TO VOCAL HEALTH

In addition to the ten voice helpers at the start of the chapter, here are several therapies that can help the voice.

PRACTICE MEASURED BREATHING

Count your breathing mentally: inhale for a count of four and exhale for a count of six. As you exhale, note how you relax your shoulders and chest. While doing measured breathing, look in the mirror and see your face and jaw relax. Now see your shoulders and neck muscles relax. Recall using all your senses when your voice sounded great, in order to replicate that good voice. Just as learning a tennis serve or a batting skill takes practice, these exercises require daily repetition.

Louisa at seventeen sang beautifully. Her teachers had always been easy going. Suddenly she was assigned to a strict teacher. I saw her to find out why her singing had become so poor. What I found were tight throat muscles. Louisa practiced the relaxation exercises and once she understood the mechanism, she was able to solve her voice problem.

When Margaret was forty-four, her voice changed significantly and she thought she must quit singing in the choir. When I tested her, her voice was excellent and I found no lesion whatsoever. I learned that she had trouble reading the music pages and was straining to read the notes. Once she obtained reading glasses and no longer strained her neck, her voice became fine again.

To repeat, your head is balanced, but you must have some front and back muscle tension to keep it balanced. While it makes no difference whether both sets of muscles pull with five pounds or forty pounds, your head stays balanced. But, at forty pounds, you are impeding the vocal muscles and are hurting your muscles, so the exercises for relaxing your throat are very important for a good voice.

Protect the Vocal Cords

For vocal cord swelling, sucking on anti-inflammatory lozenges such as Clear-ease can help. Avoid gargling, as this strains the voice. If you are in an interview and your voice is not good, try silently laughing, or better yet, say something humorous if appropriate. Also, inhaling steam with the tongue stuck out either from a basin of hot water or from a long hot shower is beneficial.

Try Voice Lessons

Going for a job interview is not the time to learn good public speaking. The time is in high school. I am not referring to great stage presence. But a clear voice that is pleasant to hear can often make a huge difference in salary and social advancement. It really takes little training to develop such a voice. There are Toastmaster's Clubs and courses via the Internet too.

Another easy way to develop a good voice is to use the voice-to-text dictation feature on the iPhone 6. You need to speak clearly and steadily to get the words printed right! "Uh-huh" and "duh" show up too! With practice your words will flow evenly, smoothly, and confidently. To use this feature, simply:

- Set the phone to an e-mail mode.

- Press the microphone button.

• Speak a sales pitch or argument in a clear tone.

   Daily practice will improve your voice.

   In the world of 2015, getting a job and keeping it depends on multiple skills. Learning to do brain surgery takes time and effort; considering how important the voice is, the time and minimal costs for good speaking can be one of the most important job skills you can have.

11

HOW TO STOP SNORING WITHOUT SURGERY

HERE ARE SEVERAL ANTI-SNORING AIDS:

- Establish a regular sleep routine and schedule.
- Clear nasal mucus and sinus congestion.
- Sleep on your side (preferably the left side if possible).
- Open your nasal passage by lifting up the nasal tip to open the airway.
- Keep the bedroom dark.
- No exciting reading in bed.
- No eating after eight o'clock at night.
- Strengthen your throat muscles.
- If you fall asleep during the day, get sleep tested. If you *ever* fall asleep while driving, get tested for sleep apnea.

Snoring occurs when your breathing is obstructed in some way during sleep. Snoring that is annoying to the partner, snoring that keeps the partner from sleeping, and snoring that is caused by sleep apnea (a sleep disorder) are all degrees of the same condition. For example, the tonsils may start to enlarge in "social" (common) snoring, get larger in severe snoring, and practically block the airway in sleep apnea. Conversely, if the blockage is due to a fatty heavy soft palate (the soft tissue at the back of the mouth) and a large uvula (the little ball hanging down from the soft palate), as the person loses weight, the palate size will shrink and the patient's condition will go from sleep apnea to simple snoring or even no snoring.

Unlike common or severe forms of snoring, which are a nuisance but not especially harmful, sleep apnea, also known as obstructive sleep apnea, is a serious condition in which the individual has obstructed breathing or quits breathing during the night. The patient may actually turn blue due to the low amount of oxygen in the blood. Such people are tired; they awaken feeling tired and often need to fall asleep during the day. Motor vehicle and industrial accidents may be the result of sleep apnea (20 percent of traffic accidents are due to poor sleep). The same factors— a thick, heavy soft palate and big uvula, enlarged tonsils and adenoids, and large tongue that falls back—all are responsible for the noisy breathing of snoring, but the difference is that in sleep apnea, the passage of air actually stops. During those periods, the brain is without oxygen and changes that affect brain function can occur.

WHY YOU NEED TO STOP SNORING

New evidence shows that sleep apnea causes hypertension and cancer! Yes, researchers report that cancer is four times higher in persons with sleep apnea. The theory is that the body makes new blood vessels to make up for the lack of oxygen. These vessels feed young cells, which happen to be the immature cancer cells, and the good circulation awakens them. That snoring increases your risk for hypertension has been reported for many years. Here, it is thought that, in response to the interrupted oxygen flow, your blood pressure goes up so that the body can get more oxygen to your brain.

The higher incidence of diabetes with sleep apnea is not well understood.

Three other health reasons why you need to stop snoring are: 1) You sleep poorly. The next morning you need energy, so you consume extra cookies. This adds fat to the uvula and throat tissues so you snore even more. The more fat, the more you snore. 2) Your inhalation is obstructed. To overcome this blockage your stomach pushes in and your diaphragm pushes down harder. This pushes on the stomach and pushes stomach acid from the stomach into the esophagus up into the throat. The more the acid reflux, the more the swollen tissue, the more you snore. 3) Snoring by one partner affects the good sleep (and health) of the other.

WHAT MAKES THE NOISE?

When you pluck a string of a guitar your hear a sound when that string vibrates. When you bang a drum that drum surface vibrates and makes a sound. Snoring is the noise caused by vibration during the in-breath, or inhalation. Which structure actually vibrates depends on many factors. Usually, it is the soft palate that is the weak muscle that falls back in sleep. The problem is that there are other muscles that may be "weak" or flaccid and block the airway.

Other structures may be causing the noise including the tongue, epiglottis, or throat tissue and swallowing muscles. Frequently, there are oversized tonsils or an oversized uvula that is the reason for the sound. Normally, before the in-breath, the muscles of the upper airway tighten to keep the airway open. But in sleep, that muscle tone may be reduced. Nonetheless, most people have sufficient tone in their palate, tongue, and muscles of the throat tissue to keep an open airway.

Normally, the soft palate and other muscles maintain tone so that when a person lies flat, the palate stays "up in the air" and doesn't block the airway. This is why snorers can get relief by sleeping on their side. This is also why sleep specialists recommend tying an old tennis ball on the back of a T-shirt. When you sleep on your back, you feel the ball and turn on your side. The weaker the soft palate and the more fat around it, the more it will fall back in sleep, where it can cause blockage or obstruction.

Far back in the tongue, below where you can see it, is an area of lymphoid tissue that acts like the tonsils called the lingual tonsils. Sometimes this tissue is enlarged and causes sleep apnea because the tongue falls back and the lingual tonsils push the epiglottis backward to reduce the airway. (The epiglottis is the lid just behind the tongue that closes over the windpipe to keep food from going to the lungs when swallowing.) The enlarged tissue can be seen by the specialist using a telescope or mirror.

Although enlarged adenoids are a common cause of children's snoring, it is uncommon in adults because, as a rule, the adenoids atrophy as we age. Generally, they are gone by age fourteen. If the adenoids are large enough to be obstructive in adults, a careful evaluation and probable biopsy is needed. If the obstruction in the adenoid area is on one side only, an immediate full evaluation is needed to rule out a growth.

Snoring in children is an important symptom and needs to be treated. See Chapter 16 on Kid Stuff.

COMMON CAUSES OF SNORING

- Structures in the throat such as adenoids that block breathing.

- Soft palate and uvula fall back in sleep and block breathing.

- Tongue is large or falls back in sleep.

- Structures in the lower throat and voice box that block breathing.

- Any excess fat that makes the soft palate and uvula heavier, causing them to fall back more easily.

- Extra fat that is deposited in the throat tissues can cause vibration and blockage.

- Nasal blockage such as from a cold, nasal polyps, or postnasal drip.

- Nasal congestion, postnasal drip, and chronic sinusitis.

- Allergic rhinitis.

IS IT SLEEP APNEA OR SOCIAL SNORING?

Do you have sleep apnea or just common social snoring? Because sleep apnea has serious health consequences, your doctor may refer you to a sleep specialist who can give you a sleep apnea test (more on this in a moment) to help differentiate between the two. Social snoring may not cause dangerous changes in the oxygen to the body as sleep apnea does, but it is serious because it can become sleep apnea. There can be injurious social consequences. Studies have shown that when the partner who doesn't snore loses sleep, there are health consequences. Besides, sleeping on the couch or in another room is not conducive to marital bliss.

In a sleep apnea test, sleep specialists measure and record the drop in oxygen during periods where no air goes to your brain. A sleep study test is done in a special laboratory, where you can be monitored overnight as you sleep. During the test, the patient is connected to several devices such as an electroencephalogram (EEG), an electrocardiogram (EKG), and oxygen and respiration monitors. These devices are used to record the patient's brain waves, blood oxygen level, heart and breathing rates, sleep stages, and other indicators as he or she sleeps. The periods of time during sleep when the patient stops breathing are called apnea episodes. The apnea episodes are counted and compared as to frequency and severity. This tells your doctor and sleep specialist how severe the problem may be.

For most people with diagnosed sleep apnea, the first treatment doctors prescribe is continuous positive air pressure (CPAP). This approach involves wearing a mask-like device that you wear on the nose while sleeping. The mask is connected to a machine that forces air into the lungs, overcoming the uvula or other blockage. The pressurized air keeps the airway open, which decreases snoring and sleep apnea.

Other methods to clear sleep apnea and snoring include clearing the nose and sinuses, and massaging the throat tissue to reduce its size and flab. (More on these methods next.) Because excess fat in the soft palate and throat tissue is a common cause of sleep apnea, and the incidence of this sleep disorder among overweight persons is quite high, losing weight is often recommended.

LIGHTS OUT

For a good sound sleep, the room should be dark–even the red-projected time from a digital clock can be a problem. A flashing billboard sign that lights up your bedroom is a disaster. If you get up for the bathroom, do not put on the overhead light. This tells your sleep center that it is now daylight and time to get up. Use a nightlight placed low on the floor, never an overhead light.

A WHOLE BODY APPROACH TO PREVENT
OR QUIT SNORING

Whether you have social snoring or sleep apnea, let's clear the condition to prevent the bad results. In my practice I always try these simple remedies first to see if they work and to avoid the sleep apnea test, CPAP, or surgery.

Use Pulse-Wave Irrigation
to Clear the Nose and Throat

Using pulse-wave irrigation for the throat as well as the nose is an important tool for snoring. The nasal irrigator attachment is used to clear nasal or sinus blockage; the throat attachment is use to strengthen the throat tissue, reduce fat flab, and reduce size of swollen tonsils.

The tonsils may be enlarged due to infection or tonsilloliths (also known as tonsil stones or tonsoliths). These are white cheesy deposits in the crypts or holes of the tonsils. Having tonsilloliths is not a disease. The white material is simply dead bacteria and white cells. It is the tonsil doing what it is meant to do. Although a breath condition may occur, it is not a disease that requires rushing to the doctor. The throat irrigation tip is specifically designed to clear out the white material from the crypts. To reach the tonsils with the irrigator, lay the throat tip of the irrigator on the right side of the tongue and point the tip to just behind the last tooth. This automatically directs the stream to best remove the tonsilloliths. The irrigator's pulsating stream acts like a massage, bringing fresh blood to the area. This massage clears infection that may be the cause of the tonsil enlargement and resolves the extra swelling. Reducing the tonsil size will help keep the airway open in sleep. For snoring, use this throat irrigator twice a day (see page 129 for directions). With this method, there is never a need to remove the tonsils because of tonsilloliths or snoring.

If the uvula is so enlarged and extends for inches down the throat, it is best to simply snip off the excess tissue by surgery.

If there is nasal congestion or postnasal drainage, use the nasal irrigator of the Hydro Pulse device twice a day too (see page 54 for directions). The nasal-pulsing stream acts as a massage to milk away the swollen nasal tissue. This enables better nasal function and nasal cilia movement and reduces swollen nasal tissue. The combination of nasal irrigator and throat irrigator is especially effective for snoring.

SING AND EXERCISE THE THROAT MUSCLES

Speech therapists use throat exercises to strengthen the throat muscles and increase their tone. The goal is to make the throat tissue stiffer with less fat. These same exercises reduce snoring. In snoring, often the throat tissue and the soft palate are flabby. In sleep that blocks the air passage causing vibration sounds and blocking air to the brain. Forceful mouth blowing can be therapeutic. Any forceful blowing—say, through a trumpet or a didgeridoo or by inflating a balloon—will strengthen the throat muscles and reduce snoring. Routinely my patients who perform the following exercises are able to stop snoring.

It takes time to build and strengthen muscles by exercise and the throat is no exception. Do each exercise for three minutes.

- Hold the tongue on the hard palate (the bony hard palate in the front part of the roof of the mouth). Say the vowel sounds A, E, I, O, U. Move the tongue around as you do these. The sounds should be loud.

- Place the tongue in front of the roof of the mouth. Then slide it all the way to the back of the roof of the mouth while pronouncing the vowels. Pronounce the vowels rapidly.

- Press the tongue forcefully against the hard palate. Press frequently.

- Press the tip of the tongue into just behind the lower incisor teeth while pushing the back of the tongue into the floor of the mouth.

- Blow up a balloon by sniffing air in hard through the nose and forcing it out hard against the balloon with your mouth.

- Swallow keeping the tongue on the roof of the mouth.

- Repeat the words "ah hung" loudly. Feel that palate moving. Repeat this with the tongue moving around the roof of the mouth.

- Blow the didgeridoo (see page 170).

Blow the Didgeridoo

The didgeridoo is a native Australian wind instrument developed by its indigenous peoples. A university study showed that playing the didgeridoo can relieve sleep apnea in some patients. A version of this big Australian horn is available on the Internet for seventy-five dollars. It takes a lot of forceful blowing to get the sound and that strengthens the muscles and thins throat fat. Forceful mouth blowing such as through a trumpet also strengthens the throat muscles. At the same time these exercises reduce extra fat and swelling in the throat. The didgeridoo method is especially effective if you started snoring in middle age and are not significantly overweight. (See the Resources section to learn where you can find out more about the didgeridoo.)

Open the Nasal Valve

Increasing the area of the nasal passage with dilator strips is another help for snoring. Some people have weak cartilage on the sides of the nose. When they take a forceful deep breath, the sides of the nose collapse, causing obstruction and forcing them to mouth-breathe and snore. These adhesive strips help widen the nostrils and can be helpful to the individual who has flaccid or weak sides to his nose.

This was the tragic situation of Michael Jackson. In looking at his photographs, I can see the very poor nasal valve opening. Despite the cruel accusations that the press made, he did have difficulty falling asleep because of his poor airway. Based on my interpretation of his airway, this could have been a major factor in the cause of his death rather than the anesthetic propofol (Diprivan) he was given. Actually, Diprivan is considered to be a safe drug for use by anesthetists.

In some people, especially in the aged, the tip of the nose can hang down. The reason the tip comes down in age is because of a natural reduction in fat under the skin associated with aging. This depression causes the nose to block, too, by closing off the nasal valve. Simply taping the depressed nasal tip upward can open the nasal valve for air passage and solve a snoring problem. Try gently tilting the tip of the nose up to see if this improves breathing. Try tilting it up to the side, too. If you find a position that works best, run a quarter-inch strip of medical tape from just below the bottom of the nose tip, up the surface of the nose to the area of the nose between the eyes, and sleep with the nose tilted up this way. In addition to reducing the snoring, you get better sleep, too. Taping the nose up also works where the sides of the nose collapse on inhalation. Also, consider testing this out if your snoring is caused by blockage from a sinus condition or allergy.

A droopy tip can also be treated by replacing the missing fat surgically with a stent or by fixing the tip in an elevated position.

GET MOISTURE INTO THE NOSE

Many people have nasal dryness. This impairs breathing, causes unpleasant sounds, and can be a serious factor in causing snoring and other problems. Nasal dryness may cause a secondary nasal infection, crusting, and dry mouth as well. In a dry nose, the body's natural immune defenders (lysozymes and disease-fighting white blood cells) can't get to the bacteria. A dry nose can't wash out pollens and dusts. A homemade saline spray, made of 1 teaspoon of salt to a pint of water, helps. Just add to any spray bottle or device. A saline product that contains the body's natural electrolytes, such as Breathe-ease XL Moisturizing Spray, is effective in providing moisture. Also, Simply Saline is a product that contains no preservatives and is easy to carry with you; like Breathe-ease XL, there is no limit to the number of times you use it daily. Whichever moisturizer you use, just be sure that it is fresh and doesn't contain harmful preservatives or anti-caking products. A moisturizing nasal gel such as Breathe-ease XL used at night is best because it lasts much longer than saline spray.

It is important also to keep the bedroom moist. I recommend using pans of water in the room that will evaporate. This is usually sufficient. In a hotel, hang wet towels near the bed. The fancy vaporizers have been implicated in spreading allergens and mold, so I don't recommend them for daily use.

If using a moisturizer spray during the day and a moisturizing gel at night, plus taping the tip of the nose up at night, works to significantly reduce your snoring, a test for sleep apnea and the need for CPAP or surgical corrections may not be required.

SLEEP PROBLEMS AND DEPRESSION

Charles Bae, a physician in the Sleep Disorders Center at the Cleveland Clinic used a patient questionnaire to measure depression in patients with snoring and sleep apnea. He reported that depressive symptoms are shown in persons with sleep apnea. Then when they used CPAP for four hours, their depression was significantly improved. This is important to know because whatever interferes with good sleep can cause depression; therefore, instead of handing out pills for depression, a better treatment is to improve sleep.

Jay, age forty-five, was assured that he didn't snore by his partner. He got a foreign body stuck in his throat and there was considerable trauma to the throat in removing it. He was hospitalized for three days without food to allow any tears to heal.

Two months later his main complaint to me was snoring that bothered his partner. He was normal weight, had had his tonsils and adenoids out as a child, and had no nasal complaints. On examination his nose and soft palate were normal. But the soft tissue of his throat was edematous (retaining fluid). For Jay, his snoring was due to swelling of the thin lower layer of throat tissue and swallowing muscles due to his trauma. Instead of prescribing an anti-inflammatory, I recommended he first try Clearease, a lozenge that contains a mixture of the anti-inflammatory fruit enzymes papain and bromelain. You melt the lozenge in your mouth between the cheek and gums. These enzymes work to reduce the inflammation. I recommend one lozenge, four times a day. He responded to the proteolytic enzymes to reduce that swelling.

There are sleep disorders other than obstructive sleep apnea. These are best diagnosed and treated by specialists in sleep disorders who are certified by the American Academy of Sleep Medicine (see Resources section).

SURGICAL CORRECTION OF SLEEP APNEA

Surgery can be performed for snoring and sleep apnea and may be an option in some cases. The following are the most common procedures.

- Tongue-suspension procedure: Involves passing a suture through the base of the tongue and attaching it to a screw inserted into the lower jawbone to keep the tongue from falling backward in sleep.

- Pillar procedure: Involves inserting stiff stents much like collar stays into the soft palate to prevent the palate from vibrating.

- Sclerosing solution injections: Involves injecting a sclerosing solution (sodium tetradecyl sulfate) into the soft palate to cause stiffness and hardening.

- Somnoplasty: Uses radiofrequency to "cook" the tissue of the uvula and soft palate, which causes the tissue to shrink.

- Uvulopalatopharyngoplasty: Consists of using a laser to shorten the palate and remove the uvula and tonsils, thereby significantly enlarging the airway.

For surgical correction of sleep apnea, a correct diagnosis and the surgeon's surgical experience are of paramount importance. The soft palate blocks passage to the upper airway when you swallow food. If too much tissue is removed, there may not be enough remaining to perform this function and food may end up in the upper throat. It is a delicate balance between removing enough tissue to stop the blockage and leaving enough tissue to function when swallowing. Guidelines for snoring surgery, established by the American Academy of Sleep Medicine, require that a trial of CPAP be given first to relieve snoring before performing surgery.

MOUTH GUARDS

Some people benefit by the various mouth guard devices. These appliances prevent the tongue and soft palate from obstructing the airway. An accurate diagnosis of the patient's throat anatomy by an experienced provider is important for achieving a proper fit. Some of these are custom-made; some are simply molded. Not all patients are able to use these.

CONTINUOUS POSITIVE AIRWAY PRESSURE (CPAP) THERAPY

With CPAP, a mask is worn over the nose and mouth while you sleep. Then, during inhalation, air is delivered at a pressure sufficient to overcome the blocked airway. The difference between CPAP and the surgical procedures described above is that CPAP is practically 100 percent effective. Not all patients will respond to the exercises, massage, and other actions just provided. If not, and if the sleep apnea is severe, then CPAP can add years of life and better health.

It is perfectly natural to resist the idea of using CPAP. The thought of bringing a device into your bedroom and putting a mask over your face—how can anyone possibly sleep with that? "Anyway, I myself don't hear any snoring" and "Besides it reflects on my masculinity" are two common answers I hear when CPAP is recommended. I have heard 1,000 objections to using CPAP and I would need 100 pages to list them all. I always refer these people to patients who have used CPAP and now have energy, have lost weight, and are fully aware that they think better and feel better. Many tell me that they increased their income because of their increased energy. Just as important, patients will boast that their marital life has prospered since using the CPAP.

There are various companies that provide CPAP. Nearly all are covered by health insurance. The skill of the technician supplying the device is important and sometimes it takes several attempts to find the perfect fit. That is normal. What is important is that the benefits of getting proper oxygen to your brain and body are life saving and are well worth the inconvenience.

I have patients promise to give it a fair trial of one week. Usually the difference they feel is so dramatic, that they will continue the CPAP. It is important to remind the obstructive sleep apnea patient that although many of the mouth guards and the surgeries may not work, as a rule, the CPAP does work.

12

How to Recover a Loss of Smell

Some Tips on Dealing with a Loss of Smell:

- Avoid a dry nose and throat.
- Add a squirt of lemon or lime to drinking water to dispel thick mucus.
- Clear any nasal blockage.
- If the problem is just starting, see a doctor right away for treatment.
- If you have nasal polyps, get them cleared (the longer your olfactory center is blocked, the less chance for recovery).
- Practice stimulating your olfactory smell stem cells.
- Get a thorough medical checkup to rule out a systemic condition.
- Is the problem due to toxic inhalants such as formaldehyde, chlorine, etc?
- Is it the medicine you are taking?
- Install smoke detectors and gas leak detectors in your house.

Peter used a zinc spray to help clear the congestion in his nose and immediately noticed a loss of smell. He saw me that same day and I placed him on systemic prednisone (a corticosteroid medication), as well as a cortisone nasal spray to go directly to the olfactory (smell) area. He was able to regain his sense of smell.

The ability to smell comes from sensory nerves that project from the top of the skull through tiny holes in the ethmoid bone, a bone that separates the nasal cavity from the brain. The nerves end at the upper third of the nose, both on the central septum side and on the lateral (side) walls of the nose. An odor gets to the upper third of the nose and enters a cup-like nerve ending. The smell particle dissolves in this cup structure and the composition creates an electric current the travels up through the openings in the ethmoid bone, where it is then transmitted to the olfactory bulb organ. From there, the message can be transmitted to emotional or stress areas of the brain. When you smell a lover, it sends a message to the pleasure center; when you smell a tiger, that sends a message to the fight-or-flight center.

One pleasure of mankind is the sense of smell. In the embryo the olfactory organ is the first and largest cranial nerve to form. At the roof of the nose, there are projections from the olfactory nerve that descend from the brain through tiny openings right into the nose. At the end of the nerves are receptor cells that tell the nerve whether the smell is something dangerous or pleasant.

Volumes have been written about the pleasures of smell and no wonder. The olfactory sense is connected to the limbic system, the emotional center of the brain. In my local shopping mall, there are at least three outlets that cater to perfumes for attraction and aromatherapy. Pheromones are the odors that are given off by many female mammals for sexual attraction and stimulation.

Our sense of smell is one of our main protectors against danger and disease. Thanks to it we can quickly run when we smell something dangerous and avoid spoiled food without ingesting it.

TYPES OF SMELL IMPAIRMENT

There are varying degrees of loss of smell. Here are the different forms:

- *Anosmia* refers to having no sense of smell at all.

- *Hyposmia* refers to having a reduced or partial sense of smell.

- *Parosmia,* also known as troposmia or cacosmia, is an olfactory dysfunction that is characterized by the inability of the brain to properly identify an odor. It is a distorted sense of smell. For example, usually the receptor cell for perfume goes from the nose to the olfactory smell section in the brain that identifies perfume. In parosmia, the person identifies perfume as burnt rubber. There are several theories to account for this: One is that the receptor cell for perfume has somehow gotten the wiring mixed up and instead goes to the brain receptor for burnt rubber; this is very difficult for the patient since there is no objective evidence to prove his or her claim that spoiled meat smells like perfume. This is similar to referred pain, such as when heart pain is felt as pain in the hand or neck pain is felt in the area above the eye.

- *Phantosmia* is a form of olfactory hallucination; it is the perception of odors when there is no odor present. This is different from misidentifying perfume as smelling like rubber. Phantosmia can occur in migraine headaches and also in pregnancy; fortunately, it is transitory. Some people have responded to taking venlaxine (Effexor), a serotonin-norepinephrine reuptake inhibitor that is used to treat depression and other conditions such as anxiety and nerve pain.

WHAT CAUSES A LOSS OF SMELL?

Anosmia refers to the loss of a sense of smell. The most common cause of ansomia is a virus that attacks the olfactory nerves and causes them to swell. Because the nerves are in very narrow bony openings, the swelling cuts off their circulation and causes the nerves to die. During the polio epidemic of the 1930s, it was found that the poliovirus entered the brain via these olfactory openings and attempts were made to close these openings to prevent the polio disease. But when those openings were closed with zinc spray, the sense of smell was lost.

As one of the five primary sensory organs, a loss of smell can cause significant handicaps. Your sense of taste is altered because when you taste food, what you taste and enjoy is made up of both taste and smell. Try to enjoy a delicious steak with your nose plugged. You won't really taste it, much less enjoy it. With a cold, your sense of smell and taste are both affected.

Any infection such as a sinus infection or trauma to the olfactory area can cause the nerve fibers to swell, because the nerves go through very narrow canals from the olfactory center to the end of organs within the nasal chamber. A direct fist blow to the nose may transmit to the ethmoid bone, where the nerves are located. Ethmoid bone trauma can cause nerves to swell. Surgical trauma can do this too.

Whatever blocks the pathways to the olfactory nerves can cause anosmia. A loss of smell can follow from a bout of acute sinusitis, the common cold, allergic rhinitis, or influenza. A deviated nasal septum, nasal polyps, and allergic swelling will block access of the smell particles to the olfactory sensors. Changes in brain function are a cause of anosmia. In Alzheimer's disease, anosmia is an early symptom. Anosmia is seen in those with diabetes, malnutrition, and deficiencies of thiamine and zinc. Huntington's disease, Parkinson's disease, schizophrenia, and dementia are also associated with anosmia. It is normal for our sense of smell to decline in old age.

Head injuries, even without skull fracture, are a cause. This is especially true if the brain is moved about enough to strain the olfactory nerves. It is seen in boxers. Recent studies show that concussion, especially repeated athletic concussions, reduces the ability to identify smells.

Direct trauma to the olfactory bulb may include tumors, aneurysms, radiation to that area, and stroke.

Localized nasal membrane changes include tissue atrophy (atrophic rhinitis) and Sjögren's syndrome with dry mouth and eyes. Inhaling chemicals such as cocaine, solvents, and printing powders will also damage the membranes.

Camille came to me in panic: she couldn't smell her cooking or perfumes. I could not find a nasal cause and had her go for a complete physical. They discovered she had diabetes, corrected it, and her sense of smell improved.

Anosmia can occur if any part of the nerve pathway from the smell receptors in the nose to the brain are damaged. Clearly, the causes of anosmia are many:

- Aging

- Alzheimer's disease

- Certain over-the-counter nasal sprays with zinc

- Chronic allergies
- Common cold
- Complications of nasal or sinus surgery
- Cystic fibrosis
- Drug side effect
- Endocrine disorders
- Excessive smoking
- Head trauma
- Heavy nose blowing
- HIV infection
- Huntington's disease
- Liver disease
- Nasal growths or masses
- Parkinson's disease
- Recreational drugs (cocaine)
- Rhinosinusitis
- Sarcoidosis
- Toxic gases such as toluene, chlorine, or toxic vapors
- Uremia/dialysis
- Viral infection
- Wegner's granulomatosis
- Work-related toxic substances (Skydrol)

Loss of smell is ordinarily due to a viral infection; however, it may also signal a specific medical condition that needs treatment. If you are using a new nasal spray, I recommend that you test your sense of smell before using the new spray. That way, if this product does affect your sense of smell, you will recognize it right away and get treatment.

Where difficulty in smelling is due to nasal blockage, it is advisable to correct that blockage. In theory, the longer the olfactory area of the nose is blocked, the more the nerves will atrophy from disuse. This may mean clearing nasal polyps that block the airway, or straightening a deviated nasal septum that is blocking breathing, or clearing a chronic sinus condition.

Loss of smell is tested by having the patient try to recognize known odors. One common test uses rose, orange, peppermint, leather, and fish. The Anosmia Foundation has a listing of common smell tests and their differences. Many of these include scratch-and-sniff tests that you can do yourself (for more information on smell testing, see the Resources section).

A WHOLE BODY APPROACH
TO IMPROVE YOUR SENSE OF SMELL

The ability to enjoy pleasant smells is an important part of the joy of living. Let's preserve it—or better still—let's enhance it.

CLEAR YOUR NASAL CONGESTION AND ANY SINUS INFECTION

If the loss of smell occurs with a cold, an allergy, or a sinus infection, it will typically resolve when the original condition is cleared. Use a corticosteroid nasal spray such as Flonase daily. Note that the organ of smell is in the roof of your nose between your eyes. When you use the spray, drop your head onto a pillow and imagine you are trying to get the drops to go through the nose, through the top of your head, to the floor. Try to remain in this position several minutes, but be careful not to strain your neck. Be sure to use a pillow or appropriate support.

TAKE A VITAMIN B6 SUPPLEMENT

Ask you doctor about taking vitamin B6 (pyridoxine). I advise taking 100 milligrams twice a day. Pyridoxine is an important part of the neural chemistry and has been found useful in many nerve conditions.

USE SMELL-RECALL EXERCISES
TO GROW NEW OLFACTORY CELLS

The olfactory area is a rich source of stem cells. In theory, stem cells in the olfactory areas can be stimulated to grow new nerves for smell. The evidence for this is that some individuals, who have lost their smell sense, get it back. Although there is currently no proven means of directing these stem cells to produce olfactory cells, I have a method that may work.

My approach is to have patients take a lemon, hold it under their nose, and actively recall what it smells and tastes like. Or use any favorite perfume or lotion. This exercise has worked for some patients. Recently, I read a book by a chef who taught cooking. She lost her smell sense from a viral infection. She described how she managed to continue teaching by carefully measuring cooking recipes. Daily, she looked at the cinnamon and figured out the proper amounts. Her taste was intact so she could taste salty or sweet and sour. Eventually, her smell sense did return, although not as acute as it was before. With the constant stimulation of food odors—she would see the product and her mind recalled the smell—apparently, her stem cells grew new olfactory cells. Do the smell-recall exercise for at least fifteen minutes a day.

The positron emission tomography (PET) scan is a significant aid to understanding how the brain works. The brain uses glucose for food. By having a person take a prepared radioactive glucose that can be detected in the brain by the tomography, doctors can tell if a strong smell is being metabolized in the olfactory area. In one study of eleven patients who developed anosmia following a virus, there was less metabolism in the amygdala region of the brain, where smell is perceived.

Whether doing the smell-recall exercise above stimulates the stem cells in the smell organ or builds up new brain connections so that smell is perceived, there appears to be two mechanisms that contribute to repairing the anosmia:

1. Neuroplasticity shows that new circuits can be created in the brain. Just as stroke patients can regain their loss of speech, daily repetition of smelling and recalling favorite odors encourages both venues in people with loss of smell.

2. Stimulation of the stem cells may create new brain connections. It is important to do the smell-recall exercises for at least fifteen minutes a day. Now that we know that the brain areas show less function and that new brain circuits can be formed, there is more reason to recommend smell-recall exercise.

ENHANCE YOUR SENSE OF SMELL

To keep young, doctors recommend mental exercises. Because the sense of smell can diminish with age, practices for improving that sense can be quite useful. Try recognizing odors. Practice identifying cooking odors

PLAY IT SAFE

If you have lost your sense of smell, take the following precautions:

- Install a gas or propane leak detector and fire alarms. Make sure the batteries in the devices are kept active.

- When cooking, check the oven and stovetop periodically to make sure nothing is burning.

- Label and date perishable foods and keep them refrigerated. Throw them out when they have expired so you don't accidentally eat a food that has gone bad.

- Ask a close friend to check your house for odors you can't detect such as mold.

---

by what is being baked. Have someone test you on your own lotions and perfumes and study getting them right. At the store perfume counter, test the sample before you find out the contents. Can you recognize jasmine? Practice picking up odors related to objects—clothing, flowers, and others. Visit the gardening section and practice recognizing the odors of the various flowers. The sense of smell identification can be developed like a stronger muscle. As your sense of smell develops, you will learn to identify cloth, wool, and so on through practice. Learn to recognize wines, inhale the wine and see if you can recognize it next time. Use your smell to identify spoiled wine. Enlarging your sense of smell recognition is a boost for your brain. Use this smell enhancement method for fifteen minutes a day.

In a 2014 study of more than 3,000 older Americans, researchers found those who were unable to detect scents such as rose, orange, peppermint, leather, and fish were more than three times as likely to die in the next five years, compared to those with a sharp sense of smell. The study reported that those with the sharp sense of smell who identified four out of the five smells were more likely to be alive in five years. Although many factors such as diabetes, hypertension, and others might account for the difference, why not improve your sense of smell as a potential aid to overall health?

The MRI scan has been a significant aid for showing changes in the brain in patients with anosmia. An MRI can show the size and shape of the olfactory bulb in the smell center. It can identify atrophy or shrinkage of the organ as well as its re-enlargement. Would performing smell enhancement also strengthen the overall brain health? Perhaps the answer is yes.

13

HOW TO LIMIT THE HEALTH EFFECTS OF SMOG, FIRES, AND VOLCANO GASES

A FEW TELLTALE SIGNS THAT ENVIRONMENTAL IRRITANTS MAY BE AFFECTING YOU:

- Coughing
- Decreased mucus secretion
- Eye irritation
- Sinus congestion
- Sore and dry throat
- Wheezing

ENVIRONMENTAL EXPOSURES

With our current changing climate and the growing frequency of weather extremes like heat waves, droughts, floods, and fires, we are exposed to increasing amounts of harmful chemical gases and smog-forming pollutants. People exposed to these chemical compounds often experience a combination of nasal, sinus, and bronchial problems. It is important to know how these affect the respiratory system and what you can do to protect your airways.

WILDFIRES

In areas prone to drought, large-area brush and forest fires are not only becoming more frequent but are also occurring closer to populated urban areas. The smoke from wildfires is a combination of combustion chemicals such as carbon dioxide (CO_2) and burn particles. You can see the soot on your skin; unfortunately, you are inhaling those same particles unless you are properly masked.

Wildfires generally produce particles that are 0.3 microns or larger. The larger particles are too big for cilia to move out of the respiratory tract; therefore, they can cause more symptoms.

SMOG

The effects of smog on the respiratory system include cough, phlegm, runny nose, sore and dry throat, sinus congestion, wheezing, eye irritation, and bronchitis. Sulfur dioxide (SO_2) is a main component of smog and can be harmful, even when present in small amounts. Sulfur products combine with other chemicals in the air, including automobile and smokestack emissions and chimney gases, to form byproducts that can be especially harmful to people and animals. With new products being burned, dozens of new chemicals have been reported—none of which are desirable. Sulfuric acid, a very strong corrosive acid, is one byproduct SO_2 can form. No wonder your eyes burn in bad smog!

Sulfur products also act on the cilia of the nose and inactivate them. This is why your nose feels very dry and irritated on a smoggy day. Without normal cilia action to remove bacteria and dust, the bacteria multiply to cause sinus infection. In addition, the toxic products swell the sinus openings and block the sinus cavities, making an ideal medium for bacteria in sinus cavities to flourish. These harmful products also inhibit bronchial cilia, which therefore cause you to cough. (When bronchial cilia can't remove particles, then coughing takes over.)

In the killer London smog of December 1952, many of the deaths were reactions to the products formed by the smog chemicals. At that time coal was used daily for heating furnaces and fireplaces and for generating power to factories and power plants. Coal is high in sulfur compounds. The particularly cold air that month kept the chemicals from rising. Medical reports in the following weeks estimated that 4,000 people had died prematurely and 100,000 more were made ill because of the smog's effects on the human respiratory tract.

When you are stuck behind a diesel bus or truck on a smoggy day, you not only inhale CO_2 but also various combinations of SO_2 with combustion elements. When you live next to a busy freeway, you and small children will be exposed to more noxious fumes. These exposures to various fumes also occur from large-area forest fires.

FILTER MASKS: GET A GOOD FIT

Effective masks are technically called filters. Although these filters look like paper masks, they are designed to filter out 95 percent of particles that are 0.3 microns or larger. Look for a NIOSH-rated 95 filter mask. This tells you that the mask has been tested by the National Institute for Occupational Safety and Health (NIOSH) and has been shown to keep out at least 95 percent of all tiny airborne particles. The big problem with these masks, however, is that they must be fitted properly to be effective. There should not be a gap between the mask and the face that allows air to come in; there must be a good seal. A simple, loose-fitting mask will do little to combat pollution and block tiny particles. Unfortunately, most people find these masks uncomfortable and don't use them properly. Note: The ordinary dust masks for house-cleaning or the so-called surgical masks do not provide adequate filtration.

VOLCANO GASES

Volcanic eruptions such as those in Pompeii (79 A.D.) and at Mount St. Helens (2008) can be huge. Even when volcanoes are not spewing hot lava, some give off CO_2, SO_2, and other harmful gases that can slow nasal and chest cilia. If you live downwind from Kilauea, an active volcano on Hawaii's Big Island, that can be a problem, as with any active volcano. In addition to Kilauea, Mauna Loa and Lothi are active volcanoes in the Hawaiian chain There are also several active volcanoes in the United States mainland as well. However, because the Big Island is non-industrial, there are fewer toxic sulfur products than if these emissions were to take place in a city. The volcano eruption in Mount Ontake on the Japanese island of Honshu on September 27, 2014, is a reminder of the devastation that volcanoes can cause.

Signs of toxicity from sulfur fumes include a feeling of dryness in the nose and cough. After smog or volcano exposure, a cough may be due to slowing of the chest cilia. When the cilia of the bronchial tubes no longer do their job of moving dust out of the lungs, then a cough takes over. There are other gases that may be harmful from volcanoes, depending on which gases they emit. The worst volcanoes are those that emit chlorine, one of the most toxic of the possible gases.

In the 2010 eruption of Eyjafjallajökull volcano in Iceland, the main health threat was the size of the ash particles. People with pre-existing respiratory problems were mostly affected. Some people developed asthma and bronchitis; those with existing asthma or chronic obstructive pulmonary disease (COPD) experienced an exacerbation of their symptoms.

In the television mini-series *Ring of Fire* that aired in 2012, an area called the "Ring of Fire," an arc of volcanoes encircling the Pacific Ocean, demonstrated the extremely wide areas of this planet where volcanoes exist and where volcano gases affect the population. One thing was made clear: it is not possible to evacuate all the potentially active volcano areas.

A WHOLE BODY APPROACH TO PROTECT AGAINST HARMFUL ENVIRONMENTAL EXPOSURES

If you live in an area where you are exposed to smog, volcano gases, or smoke from wildfires, the following actions will help you to limit your exposure and thereby protect your nasal passages and respiratory airways.

AVOID EXPOSURE IF POSSIBLE

Reduce exposure to these harmful airborne chemicals whenever possible. Pay attention to local air quality reports. When you are stuck behind a diesel bus or truck on a smoggy day, drive with your windows up and recirculate the air. If you live next to a busy highway, keep your windows and doors closed, and use an air conditioner when it's hot outside.

USE A FILTER MASK WHEN NECESSARY

Be sure to purchase a mask that is marked N95 and that is proven to filter out 95 percent of airborne particles (see page 186). Do not rely on the paper dust masks that are commonly sold at hardware stores. These masks are designed to trap large particles such as sawdust and will not protect your nose, sinuses, and lungs from smoke. Also protect the eyes with frequent use of a soothing eye drop.

USE PULSE-WAVE IRRIGATION

Irrigate the nose once or twice a day when pollution levels are high or after exposure to environmental irritants to restore the nasal cilia. To the 16 ounces (500 ml) of saline solution, add one teaspoon of Johnson's Baby Shampoo to help remove volcanic ash, soot, and other dust particles. (For complete directions, see page 54.) It is important to restore the nasal cilia as quickly as possible to prevent complications such as chronic sinus disease.

HUM

In a low tone, say "oooommmm." Humming—like a low-pitched "oooommmm" is a vibration, not unlike the pulsing irrigation, that vibrates the cilia to help restore good ciliary activity. This is especially useful for the cilia in the chest.

DILUTE ABSORBED CHEMICALS
WITH COPIOUS AMOUNT OF LIQUIDS

Drink plenty of water along with warm or hot (not iced) green or black tea, with or without caffeine. Large amounts of these fluids help the cilia remove the toxins, which are then flushed out of the body. The larger amounts of liquid help dilute the absorbed chemicals.

KEEP NASAL PASSAGES MOIST

It is extremely important to treat dryness in the nose. The nose is supposed to moisten inhaled air to help maintain a moist environment for the cilia. Moisten the nose with a saline moisturizer spray or gel such as Breathe-ease XL or Simply Saline. Or prepare your own using one teaspoon of salt to 16 ounces of warm water. A moisturizer spray should be used three to four times a day to keep the nose moist; the moisturizer gel can be used at night.

OTHER HELPFUL HINTS

If your cough persists, it means that the cilia of the chest are not doing their job. Drink more fluids until your urine turns light. Do not use a cough suppressant because that will keep the irritants in your lungs. Instead use an over-the-counter product containing guaifenesin (Mucinex) to relieve the chest congestion. Inhale steam, for example, while taking a shower or sitting in the bathroom with the shower running. Simply stick out your tongue and inhale the steam. Consult your doctor about using an Albuterol inhaler if necessary; this bronchodilator will relax the muscles in the airway and increase airflow to the lungs.

14

HOW TO RESOLVE OTHER NASAL- AND SINUS-RELATED CONDITIONS

There are other conditions besides infection and bacteria that can play an instigating role in nasal and sinus problems. Rebound from nasal sprays, thinning of the nasal tissue, a deviated nasal septum, and nose-bleeds are just some of the common conditions that require the "gentle" skills of an otolaryngologist.

ATROPHIC RHINITIS

This unpleasant condition is called atrophic rhinitis, referring to atrophy, or thinning out of the membranes. In this condition, the nose is dry and no longer moistening the airway, and there are heavy crusts, commonly referred to as "boogers." Some people get atrophic rhinitis, by constantly picking their nose. Recreational drugs may thin the membranes so excessively that bleeding and even exposure of the bone and cartilage can occur. When the membranes thin out so that they become as thin as a single page, an individual feels uncomfortable, complains of a burning sensation in the nose, and has frequent nosebleeds. Infection is present because the cilia function is impaired. Clearing the infection may bring back the cilia function. Systemic antibiotics are not the correct treatment, however.

Proper treatments include moistening the nasal passages. Breathe-ease XL Nasal Spray (or a similar moisturizing spray) should be used three to four times a day to keep the nose moist. A moisturizing gel such as

SYMPTOMS OF ATROPHIC RHINITIS

- Frequent, minor nosebleeds

- Heavy crusting in the nose

- Boogers

- Reduced sense of smell

- Dryness in the mouth due to dry nose

- Awareness of a bad odor from the nose

- Changes in the sinus cavities

Breathe-ease XL Nasal Gel to use at night is beneficial. By moisturizing, this gel helps natural immune system healers like lysozymes get to the infection. Prescription medicines such as Bactroban ointment can also be of benefit for certain types of infectious organisms and Premarin (estrogen) vaginal cream may be effective in thickening the membranes.

Can the nasal membranes return to normal after having atrophic rhinitis? To find out, it can help to measure the nasal cilia. This is an easy test to do. Simply place a particle of saccharin in the nose and measure how long it takes for the cilia to move the particle to the throat, where it is tasted. If it takes thirty minutes or more for the saccharin particle to pass from the nose to the throat, a return to normal cilia function is not usually seen. (For other methods used to measure the cilia, see page 67.)

Larry, age thirty-seven, is a printer, who complains of nasal dryness and frequent infections. When he came to my office, he brought a big bag of the various cortisone and other sprays that he had used. His nose showed very thin membranes and crusting. His cilia system was poor because the ink powders he inhaled affected his cilia function. His therapy was to wash out his nose at work after he mixed the ink powders. With pulse-wave irrigation, his cilia function eventually returned.

CYSTIC FIBROSIS

Cystic fibrosis is a potentially life-threatening hereditary disorder. In this condition, there is an increase in the salt outside the cell wall, which causes thick sticky mucus to accumulate. This heavy mucus in the nose and chest prevents cilia movement and results in many infections in the sinuses and the lungs. People with cystic fibrosis also have digestive difficulties.

People with cystic fibrosis require antibiotics more often than normal and at higher doses. Terence Davidson, a former ENT surgeon at the University of California–San Diego School of Medicine, did much to help by innovating the use of antibiotics with pulse-wave irrigation for these patients. The pulsation makes up for the absent cilia movement, and delivers the antibiotic into the sinuses. By delivering the antibiotic directly this way, he often avoided the need for systemic antibiotics.

NASAL BLOCKAGE TO BREATHING

There are many causes that block breathing. Any nasal or sinus infection can block breathing. Enlargements in back of the nose, such as enlarged adenoids in children, can block breathing. If the tip of the nose hangs way down, it can shut off the nasal valve.

CAUSES OF BLOCKED BREATHING

• Allergy	• Enlarged tonsils
• Depressed nasal tip	• Enlarged turbinates
• Deviated nasal bones	• Foreign body
• Deviated nasal septum	• Nasal polyps
• Enlarged adenoids	• Sinusitis

Often blocked breathing is caused by a nasal septum that is deviated far to one side. The blocked side is the convex side; the opposite side is cave-shaped or concave. The concave side is roomier than the convex side; yet, the patient may says that the concave side is the blocked side. This is because, to compensate for the empty space of the concave side, the body generates an enlarged inferior turbinate, which may fill the concave side. If the septum is corrected by surgery, usually the doctor will reduce the size of the enlarged turbinate to make sure that the airway is adequate.

If the cartilage that widens the nasal openings is weak, the sides of the nose may collapse on inhalation. This situation can follow excess removal of cartilage from the sides of the nasal tip during plastic surgery to narrow a nose. For breathing impaired by the sides of the nasal opening collapsing, Breathe Right Nasal Strips work well by pulling the sides open.

BIOFEEDBACK EXERCISE FOR THE NOSE

Biofeedback is a technique you can use to learn to control your body's functions. With biofeedback, you're attached to electrical sensors that help you receive feedback about your body's functions, such as your heart rate and pulse. This technique can be used for the nose too. The nose contains nerves and blood vessels and is sensitive to various chemical and nerve stimuli.

You could purchase a $10,000 gadget that measures nasal temperature and turbinate swelling, and that will help you lower the temperature to shrink the turbinates. But if you're short $10,000? No problem. Instead, take an eraser-tipped pencil. Use a pin to stick a feather onto the end of the pencil. Hold the feather so it is moved by your nasal respiration. Try to move the feather with your nasal breathing. If you are relaxed, your body will see what to do the right way and actually open the nose so you can move the feather fully.

Here's another method: cut a piece of paper in the shape of a T, about one-half inch wide. Using some tape, adhere the top of the T to your forehead so that the long tail of the T hangs down in front of your nose. If your nose is stuffy, no air will move the paper as you exhale. As your nose opens, the paper will move farther and farther out with air from your open nose. This only works if you are relaxed—breathe in for a count of four, and out for a count of six—so your body can use its "wisdom" to follow the "thought."

This is feedback. You are feeding back to the body that when it does X, the paper moves fully. When the body does Y, the information is fed back that it is doing it wrong. As more and more correct responses come back, the body soon is doing it right. This is feedback to your autonomic nervous system, which controls the vascularization of your nose.

ORAL-ANTRAL FISTULA

An oral-antral fistula occurs when there is an opening from the mouth into the maxillary sinus. Anatomically, sometimes the root of an upper back tooth extends far into the sinus cavity. Extraction of that tooth is complicated because it may leave an opening from the mouth into the sinus cavity in the cheekbone. If the membrane that separates the tooth from the sinus breaks down before the opening has a chance to heal and it remains open, then food and bacteria from the mouth can enter the sinus and cause serious maxillary sinus disease. It is a serious complication because bacteria from the mouth get into the sinus and cause infection. Today, most oral surgeons are able to prevent this complication.

An oral-antral fistula can also occur from sinus disease itself. In this scenario, a cyst or a mass in the sinus cavity may erode the bone and create an opening into the mouth.

Either way, surgical closure must be done as soon as possible.

NOSEBLEEDS (EPISTAXIS)

Epistaxis, or bleeding from the nose, is a common complaint. Winter comes with nasal dryness and bloody noses. Let's avoid them this year! People who live in the desert don't get nosebleeds. Why do they get them in Chicago? Because in the desert, the body is adapted to the dry conditions, just as we adapt to humid conditions. But in Chicago, there are extreme changes of temperature, plus very rapid changes from very cold to very hot and dry. The poor nose can't keep up. If you do get a nosebleed, here are some suggestions I give to my patients.

To prevent nosebleeds in winter, keep a pan of water in the bedroom. Have plants in the room that take a lot of water. If you are traveling, hang wet towels in the bedroom and fill the bathtub. If you see that the water evaporate in two hours, you know that the air is too dry! Breathe-ease XL Nasal Moisturizer Gel is useful, as mentioned previously. No prescription is needed, and it is often available at airport counters where it is used by travelers to prevent nosebleeds and colds while flying. The gel is water soluble, so there's no concern of its lodging permanently in the lungs like water-insoluble products. Whichever nasal gel you use, be sure that it is water soluble. (If the gel isn't water soluble, it may drip into the lungs and remain there.)

If you are susceptible to nosebleeds, regular use of Breathe-ease Nasal Moisturizer Gel, twice a day, helps prevent epistaxis. I recommend using the gel twice a day for two weeks after the bleeding has stopped. Bactroban antibacterial ointment can also be used in this manner. It is primarily a topical antibiotic that requires a prescription and helps clear infections associated with nosebleeds. It may be prescribed by your doctor after the bleeding has stopped. Neosporin antibiotic ointment is also useful, but more people are showing sensitivity to this product, and it is not soluble for nasal use. Breathe-ease XL Nasal Moisturizer Gel is specifically designed for nasal use and provides a direct in-the-nose applicator that makes it easier to apply.

Other helps for nosebleeds include vitamin C and bioflavonoids. Bioflavonoids are natural substances found in teas (particularly black, green, and oolong) and in bananas, dark chocolate, cocoa powder, and all citrus fruits. These natural substances help strengthen the blood vessels, as does rutin, a bioflavonoid that is often successful in removing the dark skin spots seniors get.

In addition to winter dryness, there are dozens of other causes of epistaxis that physicians must consider. These include hypertension and the use of drugs and herbs, including ginkgo biloba, that thin the blood. People on Coumadin and other blood thinners should be diligent about keeping their bedroom moist and their nose moist too. Stick to using pans of water or plants that drink lots of water, rather than a vaporizer. Vaporizers may moisten the air too much and bring on an increase in dust mites, as well as destroy the wallpaper.

Winter or summer, certain medications such as aspirin or aspirin substitutes, including non-steroidal anti-inflammatory drugs, can lead to a nosebleed. The common daily baby aspirin is not a concern, unless it is combined with other similar products plus ginkgo. Some antihistamines can dry the nose excessively and there are numerous drugs for heart and other conditions that have a nasal-drying effect. Before stopping a medication, see if you can maintain nasal moisture adequately, starting with water in the bedroom.

A nosebleed with a sinus infection may indicate a certain kind of bacteria that requires an antibiotic, or it just may be from the nose being so raw from blowing too hard.

Recreational nasal drugs are significant causes of nosebleeds. Cocaine will cause the blood vessels to clamp shut, cutting off circulation and leading to ulceration and nasal bleeding. Cocaine use is a frequent cause of a hole (perforation) in the nasal septum.

Certain industrial chemicals lead to thinning of the membranes and subsequent epistaxis. Chromium and nickel are two examples. Workers in chromium mines or who do sanding are prone to symptoms. Various paint solvents and thinners are common causes. If you experience burning when exposed to chemicals in the workplace, consider washing out your nose after exposure to remove the products.

Use of various cortisone nasal sprays such as Nasarel, Flonase, Nasocort, and others may cause thinning of the membranes over time and lead to epistaxis. I have my patients alternate with the Breathe-ease XL Nasal Spray to restore the membranes so they can continue with a cortisone spray that works for them. On the other hand, cortisone nasal sprays have been used for decades with few problems; they don't cause rebound addiction.

With extreme dryness, hard crusts may form that lead to nose picking and a resultant epistaxis. Copious use of Breathe-ease XL Nasal Spray helps clear up the dryness. This liquid not only softens the crusts but also helps restore the cilia that defend the nose.

Nasal gels work well because they remain in place and moisturize for a steady period of time. Ayr Gel and Ponaris Nasal Emollient are examples of good over-the-counter products. Breathe-ease XL Nasal Gel has the advantage of coming with an in-the-nose applicator tip, so there is no waste or mess. In addition, it liquefies at the cellular as well as the nasal level and contains xylitol, a natural sugar alternative that is used in toothpastes and candies to reduce bacterial levels. When Breathe-ease XL Nasal Gel is used, apply it twice a day for two weeks after the bleeding has stopped. Any bleeding that persists despite treatment probably has an infection as the cause.

If you have seen the doctor, been treated, and still are having nasal bleeding, you probably need an antibiotic to clear an infection that is usually associated with epistaxis. Topical Bactroban ointment is often effective. But also check: Are you taking an herb or medicine that leads to bleeding such as a non-steroidal medication? Always check your blood pressure when there is epistaxis. It is frequently an underlying cause of nosebleeds. If you are taking an anticoagulant, epistaxis may be a sign that your dose is too high.

Perforated Nasal Septum

Normally, the nose is divided into right and left sides by a divider, the nasal septum, and this maintains good airway pressure. However, if there is an opening in the septum, then the passage of air is significantly changed. Some of the air from the right nostril goes into the left nostril (or vice versa), and its normal passage to the smell sensors and to the lungs is altered. Some patients complain that they feel like they are not getting enough air. The septum is an important support for the bridge of the nose; it is like a tent pole in the middle of the tent. Without that support, the bridge of the nose may collapse, creating an undesirable cosmetic effect that also blocks good breathing. When the septum no longer supports the bridge of the nose, the lower end falls down and the nose resembles a saddle.

Septal perforations can follow nasal trauma. A fall may cause blood to accumulate under the membrane covering the septum. This blood presses the cartilage and interrupts blood flow to the area. Then the cartilage dissolves and ends with a perforation. When doctors see this blood accumulation, they immediately drain the blood to prevent this complication. If your child complains of nasal obstruction after a blow to the nose, it is very important to rule out a blood clot in the septum. Blood clots must be drained as soon as possible. Septal fractures, on the other hand, rarely require emergency therapy. If you have a child, expect a few.

Cocaine causes intense vasoconstriction. When used frequently, this interruption of blood flow to the cartilage can result in death of the cartilage and a perforation. Sometimes too much cartilage is removed at septal surgery and this too can be a cause. Usually, at surgery, the crooked cartilage that is blocking the breathing is straightened and replaced back into the septum.

Ideally, membrane from the healthy septum can be moved to the perforated area to cover the opening. Various "buttons" have been tried to fill the opening. Because of the poor circulation to the area, many procedures have a high fail rate. The best treatment is to keep the area moist with nasal gel. However, once a perforation exists, if neglected, it can expand. At a certain size, the tent pole support is lost and the bridge of the nose can fall. As described previously, this is called a "saddle nose deformity."

RHINITIS MEDICAMENTOSA

Rhinitis medicamentosa is a fancy name for being addicted to nose drops (or spray). Your nose is stuffy and you can't sleep. So you squirt a few drops into the nose and it opens beautifully. Now you can breathe and sleep. But later, the nose clogs again, worse than before, due to the "rebound effect," and you use the drops again, maybe more than the first time. At first, you only use them every twelve hours; then, every eight hours; then six; and now every four hours or more often. You know the bottle says to only use it for a few days, but your nose is really plugged unless you use the drops. Meanwhile, you feel nervous and irritable. This is the "adrenergic" effect of the drops, whether you take them orally or by nasal drops or spray.

The common nasal decongestants that can cause rhinitis medicamentosa are oxymetazoline (Afrin), phenylepherine (Neo-Synephrine), and xylometazoline (Otrivin, Inspire), but any constrictor nose drop can do this. There is evidence that it is the preservative, usually benzalkonium, that is the culprit. It seems that the oxymetazoline in Afrin shrinks the nasal tissue but that the benzalkonium irritates the tissue so that you need more Afrin. Products without benzalkonium may not cause rhinitis medicamentosa. Unfortunately, they are only available from a compounding pharmacy and are expensive.

MEDICATIONS THAT MAKE YOU PRONE TO REBOUND CONGESTION

These are the common nasal sprays that can cause this condition:

- Oxymetazoline (Afrin)

- Phenylepherine (Neo-Synephrine)

- Xylometazoline (Otrivin and Inspire)

It is easy to tell a patient to stop using these products, but the misery is quite severe, and willpower often doesn't work, even in the most strong-willed person. One solution is to give the patient a course of prednisone with an antibiotic. This combination of medications will shrink the nasal tissues and reduce inflammation. Sometimes I add Benadryl at night to help the patient get some sleep. A gentler solution is to gradually dilute the amount of drops you are using. To do this:

1. Take the nose-drop solution and add an equal amount of saline solution or Breathe-ease XL Nasal Irrigation Solution. Label this bottle A. Use it for a week.

2. Now add an equal amount of saline or Breathe-ease solution to an equal amount from bottle A. Label this bottle B. Use this spray for a week.

3. Next remove twenty drops from bottle B, and add it to bottle C, with an equal amount of saline solution. Use this spray for a week.

4. Keep on diluting the solution each week until you stop the drops.

5. The extremely dilute nose spray with Breathe-ease XL can now be switched to regular strength Breathe-ease XL, without the Afrin or other product.

Since you are no longer getting the rebound effect, this is a preferred method, and you avoid using more drugs. The advantage of continuing with Breathe-ease XL is that it acts to moisten the nose and stimulate cilia action. In some cases, where Afrin has been used a long time, the cilia fail to resume good movement right away, and the nose may still feel as though it is stuffy. Hot tea, chicken soup, and compresses to the sinus area help. Pulse-wave irrigation is a rapid way to refresh the nose— this is important because the condition that caused the patient to over-use nose drops may still be present, and it is best to get the cilia moving properly.

I must emphasize that willpower is not the issue here. Rhinitis medicamentosa is a chemical condition caused by the rebound of the medication. Patients with rhinitis medicamentosa need assistance to quit the nose-spray habit. As long as the use of these products is limited, they will not cause an addiction. Best, of course, is not to get started. In most nasal conditions, use of pulse-wave irrigation opens the nasal airway, so that Afrin and similar products are not needed.

SICK-BUILDING SYNDROME

When many people working in a building that is a closed environment suddenly complain of allergy, sinusitis, asthma or an odd odor, it is time to investigate to see if something needs to be corrected. Is it formaldehyde?

When new carpets and furniture are installed without fresh air in a heated location, formaldehyde used in these products is released and symptoms occur. When Hurricane Katrina victims were placed in brand-new trailers during the cold weather, the trailers were heated and the sudden release of formaldehyde caused significant illnesses.

Anytime there is construction or remodeling inside a large office building, large concentrations of dust can be picked up and deposited in another office, leading to aggravation of respiratory symptoms.

In a recent study it was noted that buildings with lower humidity levels showed fewer sick-building complaints. This is because the buildings with higher humidity allow more mold growth.

PART THREE

SPECIAL SITUATIONS

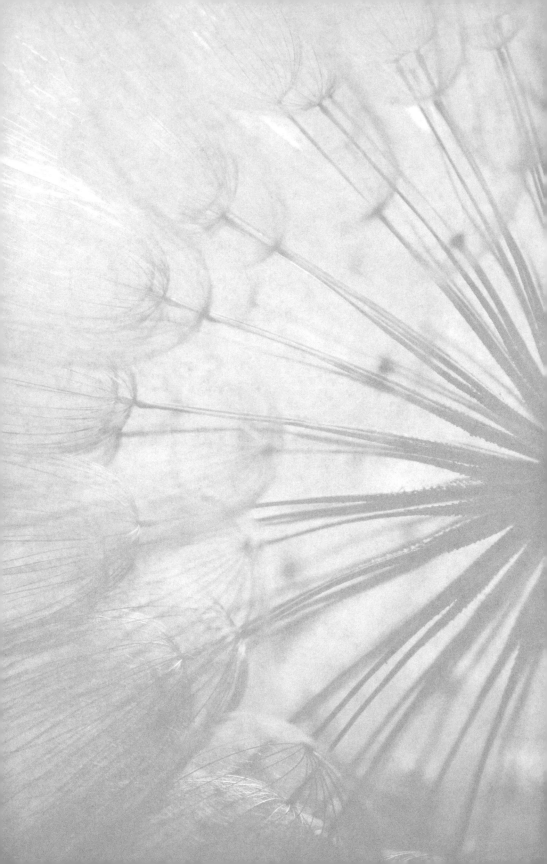

15

WHEN SURGERY
IS AN OPTION

SOME DEFINITIONS OF SURGICAL PROCEDURES
FOR THE SINUSES AND NOSE

- Balloon sinuplasty: Procedure for the treatment of blocked sinuses that involves inserting a small balloon into the sinus opening and then inflating it to force the swollen tissue open.

- Endoscopy: Procedure that uses an endoscope, which can be inserted directly into the nose without incising the skin, to examine the nose structure and passageways for any irregularities.

- Ethmoid implant: Device placed in sinuses to deliver medications.

- Image-guided surgery: Technique that gives surgeon a three-dimensional view of the nasal and sinus passages.

- Rhinoplasty: Repair of the nose for cosmetic purposes.

- Septoplasty: Surgery to reposition a deviated septum.

- Sinuplasty: Any procedure that corrects a sinus problem.

- Submucous resection: Surgery to straighten a nasal septum or to remove bone from the turbinate by elevating the mucous membrane from the bone.

- Turbinate reduction: Procedure to reduce the size of the nasal turbinate.

- Turbinectomy: Removal of one or more turbinates.

With the WBA, fewer people with chronic sinusitis need to have surgery. Yet sinus surgery may be needed when efforts to clear the cavities of disease have not been successful and the symptoms of sinusitis persist. Anatomical problems within the nose can be the cause of ongoing sinus problems. In these cases, sinus surgery may be required in order to resolve a persistent sinus problem.

COMMON SURGICAL PROCEDURES

Following are the most common surgical procedures and their indications.

SEPTOPLASTY

A deviated nasal septum is a common condition that often requires surgery. Whether due to heredity or from some nasal injury, the nasal septum may no longer be located in the midline. Instead, the thin wall that divides the left and right nasal passages is pushed over so that it blocks one side. The deviation impairs the airway for that side and may also impair drainage from the sinuses. The septum is made up of cartilage and bone; the upper bony part of the septum is formed from the ethmoid bone, and the lower bony floor of the septum from the maxillary bones. The portion between the ethmoid and maxillary bones is composed of cartilage.

Logically, the side that the septum is blocking, for example, if the septum is far to the right, then that right convex side should be the side with the disease and the nasal passage that the patient complains of not being able to breath through. However, the side that is wide open, called the concave side, is the one that the patient may complain of, and may feel that he or she can't breathe through. This is because the empty space causes the body to fill that space by enlarging the inferior turbinate. Generally, the concave side has slower nasal cilia and resultant sinus and ear disease. While performing surgery to straighten and reposition the nasal septum (called septoplasty), usually the doctor will reduce the size of the enlarged turbinate to make sure that the airway is adequate.

If the turbinate blockage is due to an enlarged or deviated turbinate bone, then the bone itself is resected so that the turbinate shelf falls to the side of the nose and no longer blocks the airway (see Turbinate Reduction next).

Septoplasty can also be used to correct a caudal septal deviation. In these cases, the external end of the nasal septum (the skin between the nostrils called the columella) has a curved or incorrect shape that needs to be surgically repositioned. Sometimes you can temporarily move the columella over to the midline. I see patients all the time who complain of poor sleep because of this obstruction. If sleep is the only concern, tilting the tip of the nose up in various directions may be sufficient to open the airway. If so, place a piece of tape that is one-half inch wide on the bottom of the nose above the columella, and place the other end of the tape on the bridge of the nose to lift the tip in place for breathing at night.

Despite various measurements, the surgeon still must make a value judgment whether straightening the deviated septum will be of significant benefit. Is this deviated septum interfering with sleep? Is this a cause of recurrent infection? Have other methods to improve breathing failed? A majority of the patients I see are referred by allergists. These patients do have allergy but despite allergy therapy, they still can't breathe well and fixing the septum is indicated.

When I evaluate a patient's deviated nasal septum I ask:

- Is sleeping normal?

- Do you tire with stairs?

- Do you tire with exercise?

- Is there a headache of nasal origin? (see Rhinogenic Headaches, page 115)

- Is your headache pulsing from an outside pressure or an inside pressure like a swelling?

- How many sinus infections have you had in one year?

- Is your sense of smell normal?

- Do your have nasal allergies?

- How many cold have you had this year?

- Do you catch colds easily?

- Do your colds hang on?

No matter how crooked the septum looks, if the patient is not being bothered, then there is no benefit in correcting that septum.

John presented with a scuba diving question. I saw his deviated septum and immediately jumped to the conclusion that he needed surgery.

"Is your sleeping normal?" I asked.

"Yes, I get good sleep every night," he replied.

"Do you tire with exercise?"

"Yes, whenever I do a twenty-five mile marathon or an all-day on a bicycle race, I feel tired."

"Is your sense of smell normal?"

"Actually, it is too good. I smell things my wife misses."

"Do you get colds?"

"Yes, five years ago I had a cold."

John did not need to have his deviated septum corrected.

When a patient has too many colds, it sends up a flag. Steve came to me to have his deviated septum corrected. He had been told by one doctor that he needed surgery, and by another doctor that he didn't need the surgery. His complaint was that he caught colds frequently and as a full-time student this was a serious problem. On examination I found that his septum in one area interfered with sinus drainage. The rest of his septum was fine. He was getting a recurrent sinus infection but, because of his excellent health, they were of short duration and he cleared them in a short time. I felt that the sinus blockage from his septum was significant and should be corrected.

If a patient has nasal congestion due to an allergy to her three cats, no matter how well I correct her deviated septum, she will still have nasal congestion from her allergy. I tell her to fix the allergy and then see whether correction of the septum is needed.

TURBINATE REDUCTION

The surgeon performing sinus or septal surgery is often faced with an enlarged or blocked turbinate. If the enlargement is tissue only, in theory, the turbinate tissue should return to normal size once the sinus disease or deviated septum is corrected. But if the tissue doesn't return to normal and it continues to block breathing after surgery, then further treatment may be necessary. In order to avoid a possible second operation, it is common for the surgeon to reduce the turbinate size at the same time as the other procedure.

One approach to treating an enlarged turbinate is called submucous resection. In this procedure the surgeon elevates the mucous membrane over the turbinate bone, removes a "strut" of the bone so that the turbinate no longer projects into the nasal cavity, and then replaces the turbinate tissue. Afterward the turbinate is lying along the side of the nose instead of in the center blocking the airway. Elevating the mucous membrane from the bone to perform this surgery is enough to reduce extra circulation and the tissue underneath. Most important, the surface where the cilia are located and the glands that supply the mucus are left intact. Other methods such as simply cutting out the extra turbinate tissue or cauterizing or treating it with a laser may damage the precious cilia. When turbinate surgery is performed, it is vital to preserve the nasal cilia function in order to prevent empty nose syndrome (see below).

A SERIOUS COMPLICATION OF SINUS SURGERY: EMPTY NOSE SYNDROME

Nasal turbinates are shelf-like structures in the nasal cavity. They serve to provide moisture, warmth, and airflow for breathing, and many of the body's natural defenses against infection. A variety of different problems are associated with the turbinates: sometimes the turbinates themselves are damaged by disease and can shrivel and no longer function; in other cases, the turbinates can swell and block breathing.

Some older medical books recommend surgical removal of diseased turbinates in order to provide adequate airflow for breathing. This procedure, called turbinectomy, is a term I abhor and a surgery that should never be done! Once removed, the turbinates can no longer provide mucus, cilia, and enzymes to protect against infection. Secondary sinus infections occur regularly and may often require three or four subsequent surgeries to clear. There can be dryness, burning, chronic nasal crusting, frequent nosebleeds, and an almost constant discomfort or pain in the nose. The pain may come from the raw surface or the exposure of nerve endings or infection. All this adds up to the empty nose syndrome, or ENS, as a side effect of surgery. In patients who have had their turbinates removed, the x-ray of the nose looks empty to the doctor, hence the term, empty nose syndrome. To take a look for yourself, see the web link in the Resources section.

In addition, the ENS patient may complain of not getting enough air, yet the doctor looks in the nose and sees that it is wide open! When the blood oxygen is measured, it is normal. How can the patient complain of not being able to breathe through the nose when examination shows it to be wide open? Even though the nasal airway is wide open, a patient with ENS feels that he or she can't get enough air! What happens is similar to a garden hose. When you narrow the hose opening, the water goes out six feet; when you open the hose completely, the water dribbles at your feet. There are sensors in the nose that tells the brain about your breathing. These sensors no longer receive the input from the airflow; so as far as the brain is concerned, you are not getting air. This condition is extremely distressful. Unfortunately, there are few options for relief once the turbinates have been removed. Prevention is best. However, the following treatments are helpful:

- Keep the nose moist with saline, preferably one that stimulates cilia such as Breathe-ease XL Nasal Moisturizing Gel.

- Apply Bactroban ointment to reduce infection.

- Use pulse-wave irrigation with xylitol to mimic cilia effect, massage the tissue, and reduce infection.

- Apply Premarin (estrogen) vaginal cream to help thicken the mucous membranes.

- Consider an implant product such as AlloDerm, which can be implanted surgically to narrow the nasal chamber and to direct the flow for better airway. AlloDerm and similar products are tissues that have had their cells removed. They provide a matrix, or support, for blood vessels and new tissue cells to grow into; thus, the implant becomes a part of the body.

At times it is necessary to move the turbinates to take out diseased sinus tissue. However, this must be done so that no turbinate tissue is harmed. There are cases where the turbinates do block breathing and moving them to the side will correctly open the airway. The method of reducing the turbinate blockage should be performed so that turbinate tissue and nasal cilia function are not damaged. Dr. Steven Houser, one of the world's leading authorities on ENS, speaks of a mucosal-sparing technique when turbinate surgery is required, as a means of preventing ENS. For the latest news on corrections for ENS, check out his website at www.metrohealth.com.

SINUPLASTY AND IMAGE-GUIDED SINUS SURGERY

Pan sinusitis is one of the worst forms of chronic sinusitis. In this condition, all the sinus cavities are filled with diseased tissue. This tissue may be polyps or diseased tissue. Nasal polyps are like grapes or bags of water, and although these polyps are rarely cancerous, they cause a significant problem for the sinuses, which clean the air passing through. They cause obstruction and chronic infection to linger in the sinuses. The patient often feels tired, complains of a low-grade fever, snores, and usually doesn't get a good sleep due to the blocked breathing. A localized severe headache is commonly associated with pan sinusitis. The polyps can also put pressure on bone and cause erosion. For this reason, pan sinusitis is a common cause for sinus surgery (also called sinuplasty).

SYMPTOMS OF PAN SINUSITIS

- Pain includes frontal and cheek regions

- Localized severe headache

- Associated cough, hoarseness and wheezing

- Nasal obstruction

- Severe snoring and poor sleep

- History of weeks of antibiotic therapy without benefit

- Poor sense of smell

- Postnasal drip

- Persistent low-grade fever that doesn't respond to antibiotics

Image-guided surgery is one technique that is used in sinus surgery. This surgery is performed using a magnetized-imaging surgical instrument that can tell the surgeon in three dimensions exactly where the instrument is and whether it is too close to the eye or the brain. Prior to surgery, a special CT image is taken of the sinuses. Then, at surgery, the position of the magnetized instrument in the nose is projected on a large computer screen in three dimensions. Now the surgeon knows exactly where the instrument is and can usually work more rapidly and with greater safety.

Fortunately, most people have only a few sinuses that are diseased and require surgery. The frontal sinus is most commonly a problem because the drainage from that sinus is long and tortuous, or the maxillary sinus may be involved because of its large size.

BALLOON SINUPLASTY

Many patients with sinus disease can be treated in an outpatient procedure called balloon sinuplasty. In balloon surgery, a guide wire is inserted into the drainage path of the sinus cavity. Attached to the guide wire is a deflated balloon. When positioned correctly, the balloon is inflated and kept in place while the sinus is irrigated using a catheter. This opens the sinus drainage and allows the disease to escape through the opening. When the balloon is removed, the sinus opening should remain open because the sinus bacteria have been removed. The advantage of this procedure is that there is minimal surgery involved.

ETHMOID IMPLANTS

Recently implants have been placed in the nose that slowly discharge medications to inhibit polyp regrowth. These products look promising. Polyps will shrink if enough systemic prednisone is given; however, there are side effects. Polyps may shrink if corticosteroid sprays are used, but the distribution and timing are irregular. By using an ethmoid implant, the corticosteroid is gradually and effectively distributed for maximum effectiveness and ease. The implant itself is absorbed. For a demonstration of how this implant works, see the web link in the Resources section.

ENDOSCOPIC SURGERY

Endoscopic sinus surgery refers to surgery that is done by means of viewing the sinuses with a telescope. This telescope, called an endoscope, is a small thin tube with a miniature camera that is inserted directly into the nose. With this viewer, often projected on a huge screen for the surgeon, the anatomy and disease is clearly seen and corrected. Thanks to endoscopic surgery, it is no longer necessary to cut through skin and bone to get to the sinus disease; it can all be done through the nose.

NASAL POLYPS

Science really doesn't know exactly why brother A gets nasal polyps and his identical twin, brother B doesn't. They are thought to be allergy-related, but expert allergy management has not cleared the presence of polyps nor prevented their return after surgical removal in many patients.

Often, polyps can be shrunk by a course of oral prednisone combined with an antibiotic. The antibiotic is needed because any infection can enlarge the polyps, and there is bound to be some infection due to the blockage. The antibiotic clarithromycin (Biaxin) is often used because it has anti-inflammatory properties and is best used with the oral prednisone. Most doctors prescribe a cortisone spray to be used after the polyps shrink to prevent their regrowth. Surgical removal may be disappointing because the same factors that caused the polyps to start in the first place are still present. Fortunately, with medications, few patients with simple nasal polyps need to have surgery. It is always a source of amazement to me that the biggest polyps, even those hanging out of the nose, respond to medication therapy.

When polyps are removed as a simple office procedure, sometimes the next day the nose is filled with polyps again! What has happened is that the visible polyps were blocking the ones in the ethmoid sinuses, and when these were unblocked, they fell down and out.

Dr. Jordan Josephson, a nasal and sinus surgeon, has written extensively on nasal polyps and their treatment. In his book *Sinus Relief Now* (2006), Josephson writes: "It is very important for the patient with nasal and sinus polyps to be on continuous medical therapies. This may include various sprays, antibiotics, and antifungals and nasal irrigation, even when the patient is feeling relatively normal. There are dietary and holistic medicines that may be helpful like acidophilus. Most importantly, the patient must remember that he still has a disease, 'nasal polyps,' which needs to be taken care of even during quiet phases of his disease. As the patient with high blood pressure needs to take care of his blood pressure, despite feeling relatively well, nasal polyp-sinus sufferers need to do the same."

People with nasal polyps must avoid aspirin, salicylates, and aspirin-related products. This is because these products are known to stimulate nasal polyp activity. For a complete list of products, go to the Reye's Foundation website at www.reyessyndrome.org.

Recent studies have correlated reduced cilia movement with nasal polyps. The hope is that restoring nasal cilia by pulse-wave irrigation may reduce polyp reoccurrence.

Note: Nasal polyps have no relation to polyps of the colon and intestines. With nasal polyps there is rarely any association with cancer or malignancy, whereas there is when there are polyps in the colon.

RHINOPLASTY

Rhinoplasty refers to correcting poor nasal bone positioning. The entire nose may be displaced to one side or the other. Or the bones may extend with a "hump" that is considered unsightly by the patient. When there is a wish to correct a "crooked nose" for cosmetic reasons, the decision to do surgery is easy. When the position of the nasal bones is impairing breathing, and the patient has no interest in cosmetic appearance, then a careful evaluation is needed regarding improving nasal function.

Are the nasal bones collapsed? Elevating them should improve airway flow.

Is the nose deviated to one side? This may narrow the airway and correcting the nose, putting the bones back in place corrects the airflow.

Since insurance doesn't pay for cosmetic surgery, insurance companies are reluctant to approve nasal surgeries for airway relief and surgeons must clarify that the rhinoplasty is needed for health reasons rather than for cosmetic reasons.

A WHOLE BODY APPROACH
TO ENSURE SURGICAL SUCCESS

After any surgical trauma to the nose or sinuses, nasal cilia will slow down. For this reason surgeons often recommend that their patients use pulse-wave irrigation in order to quickly restore normal cilia function. In the past, many sinus surgeries failed because the nasal cilia continued to be too slow after surgery and the sinus infection returned. To ensure that surgery is a success, get the nasal cilia moving afterward with warm tea, humming, pulse-wave irrigation, and the other WBA methods discussed in this book.

16

KID STUFF

SOME INSIGHTS ABOUT YOUR CHILD AND HIS OR HER NOSE:

- Don't panic at every cough and cold your kid catches.

- If there is yellow-green drainage coming out of one side of your child's nose, it is probably a foreign body that needs to be removed.

- Don't overheat the bedroom; excess heat does not add to the health of the child.

- Keep the moisture level in your child's bedroom below 50 percent—anything above and it increases mold and dust mites.

- Teach your child not to blow his or her nose excessively. Hard blowing spreads bacteria from the infected sinus to the healthy one; it also blows disease into the ear.

- If your child starts to snore, it may be a sign of enlarged adenoids.

- If your think you child can't hear, have his or her hearing checked. A cochlea implant can restore hearing to most "deaf" children so that they can develop normal speech and learning.

- If your child complains of a stomach ache after eating a specific food, suspect a food allergy.

The current thinking is that children need to get a few colds and sore throats in order to build up their immunity. Children who are overtreated at every sniffle may not develop the proper immune factors and instead may be more prone to asthma, ear infections, and sinus problems. This should comfort the parent sitting up with a sick child—your child is developing good immunity!

On the other hand, children do get chronic sinusitis. They may get ear infections too frequently. It is important that children hear well. Ear infections may cause hearing loss.

COMMON CONCERNS

Here are the most common concerns that I hear from parents and the therapies that I recommend they try before referring their child to the right specialist.

CHILDREN'S SINUSITIS

Prevent sinusitis by teaching your child not to blow too strongly or excessively when the nose is congested or stuffy. The harder the child blows, the more the bacteria are shifted from the infected area to the uninfected area and into the ear. A yellow-green nasal discharge that persists for more than a week suggests acute sinusitis; three of these episodes each year suggest chronic sinusitis. In children, a chronic sinus infection is significant if it also causes enlargement of the adenoids and results in ear infections.

The suggestions given previously for sinusitis treatment apply to children too (see pages 74–87). Those who are five or older will usually accept using pulse-wave nasal irrigation. For children age three or under, consider Proetz sinus irrigation. Here the child is positioned with the head laid way back. Very dilute nose drops are placed in each nostril, after which the nasal chambers are filled with a saline solution and aspirated using a nasal bulb syringe. When you aspirate the right side, it suctions out the purulent material from both sides and then the saline solution is added again. Check with your doctor about Proetz sinus irrigation. For a demonstration of this procedure, see the web link in the Resources section.

Enlarged Tonsils

The tonsils are located just behind the last teeth inside the mouth. Tonsils may enlarge and cause discomfort as well as snoring. Because the tonsils act as filters for trapping harmful bacteria and viruses that are breathed in or swallowed, when the immune system is weak, the tonsils become especially vulnerable to infection. Young children are especially prone to getting tonsillitis. Swollen tonsils, sore throat, and pain on swallowing are some telltale signs of an infection in the tonsils.

Tonsillectomy (removal of the tonsils) is still a common procedure. However, if you remove them you are taking out an important defender. On the other hand, if they no longer act to filter infection and are causing illness, and resist treatment, then surgery is an option.

Barry's mother asks, "Barry has had a tonsil infection every year since he was six. He is now eleven and he misses school when he gets these.

I explain to Barry's mother that one bout of tonsillitis per year is not so bad. We can reduce that with therapy and I don't recommend surgery. Also, Barry may outgrow these tonsil infections at his age.

Terry's mother complains that Patricia had three tonsil infections last year and four this year. Should Terry have her tonsils out?

Here I use the analogy of the eye. If the eye is repeatedly infected and is no longer functioning, it is best to remove it to prevent the spread of infection. On examination it was clear that Terry's tonsils were no longer functioning as a filter of infection and were now more of a cause of infection. I recommended tonsillectomy.

There have been dozens of studies regarding whether there is harm in removing tonsils in children. In the main, there is no clear evidence that removing tonsils in children is harmful. In most surgeries done for the ear, the adenoids are removed and the tonsils are left behind. What is interesting to me is that when I see patients who had their tonsils removed as adults, they report that their health did improve. Like any surgical or dental procedure, there is a certain percentage of risk involved in tonsillectomy surgery.

TONSILLOLITHS AND BAD BREATH: A SIMPLE SOLUTION

Seeing white spots in the crypts, or holes, of your child's tonsils (or your own for that matter) is not a disease. The white material is simply dead bacteria and white cells. It is the tonsil doing what it is meant to do. Although a breath condition (halitosis) may occur, it is not a disease that requires rushing to the doctor. Just use the pulsating steam of the throat irrigator to remove the material. For throat irrigation, you can use any solution–plain water, hydrogen peroxide, or a dilute mouthwash (for directions, see page 129). As a rule, children as young as five are able to use the pulse-wave throat irrigation once the parents demonstrate its use. (See the web link in the Resources section for a demonstration.) A child's bad breath may also be from a sinus infection. Lastly, don't forget the dental floss!

ENLARGED ADENOIDS

Like tonsils, adenoids help defend the body against infections. Also, like the tonsils, the adenoids can become a problem if they enlarge and block breathing. The adenoids are located just behind the nasal airways at the top of the throat. They are adjacent to the openings of the eustachian tube (the tube that connects the throat to the middle ear). The eustachian tube is essential in order to equalize the pressure in the middle ear. If the adenoids close off the tube opening, it reduces the pressure in the middle ear and can cause a number of ear problems (see next).

Besides blocking the ears, enlarged adenoids can block nasal breathing. Sometimes the adenoids are enlarged this way due to infected material draining into the adenoid tissue from sinus disease. Clearing the sinus infection may allow the adenoids to shrink. On the other hand, enlarged adenoids can be a cause of sinus disease; in which case, the sinus infection won't clear until the adenoids are removed. Which came first: the sinus disease causing the adenoids to enlarge or the enlarged adenoids causing the sinuses to be obstructive? Whichever came first, the immediate treatment is to clear any sinus drainage from the nose and to use measures to reduce the size of the adenoid. Papain and bromelain lozenges may be helpful (see page 117).

In some children there is a significant distance between the soft palate and the back of the throat. In such children, if the adenoids are removed, the soft palate will no longer close on swallowing and speaking. In these patients, a careful dissection of the adenoids that block the eustachian tube openings is done and the adenoid that aids speech and swallowing closure is left behind.

When the adenoids block nasal breathing, parents will notice snoring, crankiness, irritability, and bad breath in their child. Parents really appreciate that following adenoidectomy (removal of the adenoids) their child sleeps well without snoring, is no longer cranky and irritable, and now has sweet breath.

Chronic mouth breathing from enlarged adenoids can affect face and dental formation. Adenoid facies is a condition where chronic mouth breathing has caused changes in dental and face anatomy. Consultation between doctor and dentist is helpful here. Some practitioners take an x-ray to determine if the adenoids are blocking the airway or the ears. I rarely find this necessary, and you don't want the extra radiation.

EAR INFECTIONS

An ear infection, or otitis media, is the most common cause of earaches in children. Two of the most common types are acute otitis media and serous otitis media. In the first condition, the eardrum is inflamed, swollen, and red. Fluid behind the eardrum is thick. The child has fever and pain. Sometimes the fluid breaks through the eardrum and leaks into the ear canal, perforating the eardrum. In children, this condition comes on abruptly and is usually caused by a viral infection. Where the ear infection is chronic, it may be a bacterial infection that needs an antibiotic. Expect to have at least one viral otitis media in your child.

When the doctor looks at the ear of someone with serous otitis media, he or she sees clear fluid behind the eardrum. The eardrum is not red or swollen. There is no fever or pain. If cultured, there is no bacterial growth. In this condition, the eustachian tube is blocked, a vacuum forms and fluid fills the middle ear. In theory, this simple fluid is absorbed. In practice, the mucous cells in the middle ear change to making lots of mucus and the condition may become chronic. The fluid may thicken. By opening the ear (a procedure called myringotomy) and inserting a drain tube, you eliminate the vacuum, so the mucous cells quit overproducing serous fluid.

MYRINGOTOMY IN CHILDREN

Myringotomy tubes (often called ear tubes) are small tubes that are surgically placed in a child's eardrum. The tubes help the fluid in the middle ear to flow out. The procedure is often recommended when pus bulges the eardrum, and when there is chronic fluid in the middle ear and frequent ear infections. Before inserting the tube(s), the middle ear is irrigated with saline in order to remove all the serous fluid. The saline is then suctioned out, and the tube is placed to keep the pressure in the middle ear equal to the air pressure outside the ear.

RECURRENT INFECTIONS IN THE EARS
AND EUSTACHIAN TUBES

Many children have repeated ear infections. Often this is due to enlarged adenoids (discussed above) that are blocking the eustachian tube opening or to a child who blows his or her nose too forcefully, which then blows bacteria from the nose into the ear via the eustachian tube opening.

If your child has had two or three ear infections in one year, then a doctor should carefully examine the child's ears for evidence of liquid behind the eardrum. The treatment will vary according to your doctor's findings of the fluid. For example, the child is three and the mother reports two ear infections this year. The eardrum is clear and there is no evidence of fluid. Here I would check the nose for evidence of infection.

If there is no nasal infection, I would recommend a decongestant for the next bad cold. But if the child is three, has had two ear infections, and has thin fluid behind the eardrum, I would treat the child to clear the thin fluid. I would try a course of decongestant medications and an anti-histamine at night. And if a child with the same history has fluid that is thick and an eardrum that doesn't move well when pressure is applied, and if the child doesn't respond to the decongestant and antihistamine, then I would recommend insertion of ear tubes (see page 219) and an adenoidectomy.

When children have had repeated ear infections, in my experience, it is better to perform an adenoidectomy and insert the ear tubes as soon as the condition is evident. Most of these children then have much fewer ear infections when the blockage is corrected. The reason why? As explained earlier, enlarged adenoids can interfere with the ability of the middle ear space to stay ventilated. They change the pressure of the air in the middle ear such that it is lower than the pressure outside the ear; this creates a vacuum-like condition. To fill that vacuum, the cells of the middle ear change from air-containing cells to mucous-making cells. The longer they stay this way, the more difficult it is for them to change back. Inserting ear tubes stops the mucous-making cells. Now, the pres-sure in the middle ear becomes normal and the mucous-making cells return to being air-containing cells. With the tube in the middle ear, previous vacuum factors that may have suctioned the eustachian tube openings together, allow them to remain open.

Can the child with tubes in the ear swim? As of this writing, about half of ENT doctors allow swimming but no diving.

Note: When you go to the doctor upstairs, he recommends draining the ears with tubes but not to do the adenoidectomy. And when you go to the doctor downstairs, she recommends more antibiotic therapy. Which doctor is right? Each doctor has his or her own professional expe-rience and reasons for the recommendations. Mine is that I have found adenoid blockage in children with recurrent ear infections and I want to prevent more ear problems; therefore, I do an adenoidectomy when I do drainage and tube inserts for thick fluid in the middle ear.

DELAYED SPEECH

A common visit to my office is the pre-kindergarten child who "can't talk." Usually the child has already been to the neurologist and been declared "normal." The pediatrician has found no problem either and has recommended the parents wait and see. After I assure the parents that I can find no anatomical problem and that the child has normal hearing, I try some therapies before recommending speech specialists. Here is one recommendation that usually works.

I think that toddlers who are exposed to children's songs get confused when parents sometime imitate that speech but yet speak "adult" themselves. I ask the parents to avoid children's songs and instead to teach the child a modern cowboy or popular adult song. Church hymns are good. When I began practicing in the time of Elvis Presley, children were taught "You Ain't Nothin' but a Hound Dog!" Certainly not good English, but the goal was to stimulate the brain to imitate what they hear without hesitation. I also had the kids dress in cowboy and cowgirl outfits with a kiddie guitar and encouraged them to sing, "She'll Be Coming Round the Mountain." This method proved effective and was fun for the whole family. Either parent could participate. In contrast to special voice exercises, there was no hesitation by the parents nor was there any confusion about what to do. Other siblings could participate and even help the child. Praises from friends and grandparents for the excellent singing amplified the results.

Whatever speech difficulty the child has, this is a good place to start. Once the lyrics to "She'll Be Coming Round the Mountain" are learned, they will be more attuned to adult speech. Worst-case scenario, the child grows up with a cowboy accent!

Some children have a short frenulum (the ligament under the front of the tongue that serves to keep it from extending too far). In some children the frenulum is too short and the child cannot stick his or her tongue out far. In the majority of cases, this does not affect speech and lengthening it will not improve speech.

WHEN KIDS COUGH

A 2012 study in Israel showed that honey taken straight from the jar is useful for children, ages one to six, who have a respiratory infection and associated cough. It also helped them to sleep. The theory is that the taste and cough centers in the brain are related so that the sweet taste helps suppress the cough. In addition, honey helps thin mucus and may reduce bacteria load. Note: Honey is unsafe for babies under one due to botulism spores. Although infant botulism is rare, it can be fatal so avoid using it in the child's first twelve months.

MY CHILD WON'T EAT ORANGES

When children refuse a certain food, it may be due to a food allergy. They learn, for example, that if oranges upset their stomach, not to eat them. If you suspect your child is allergic to oranges, check out the citrus foods related to oranges and see if he or she is avoiding foods with a similar composition. Avoiding foods that the child is allergic to can help the child's health.

Children may be allergic to cow's milk, as well as to soy. Peanut and shellfish allergies are serious and may require having an emergency adrenaline pen (EpiPen) handy. It is best not to force your child to eat or drink a food when they refuse and then see the allergist for evaluation and confirmation of an allergy. Food allergy served primitive man; they learned to avoid foods that were bad for them.

SLEEP APNEA IN CHILDREN

Sleep apnea is characterized by breathing that stops frequently or for prolonged periods of time during sleep. In one sense, sleep apnea in children is more significant than it is in adults. The child with sleep apnea will suffer from daytime sleepiness, behavior problems, poor school performance, developmental delay, and neurocognitive changes. He or she may develop a secondary lung pathology such as a retracted sternum that affects breathing. The child is irritable, cranky, has bad breath, and is tired. School grades plunge.

Sleep apnea in children is often caused by an obstruction in the airway from enlarged tonsils or adenoids or both. However, approximately one-third of children who undergo tonsillectomy and adenoidectomy to resolve sleep disordered breathing are not benefitted by the procedures. For this reason, a full evaluation of your child's sleep apnea should be performed before surgery to rule out allergy, sinusitis, obesity, and tongue enlargement as factors that might be eliminated before or at surgery.

One last WBA suggestion: current thinking suggests that eating yogurt and taking probiotic supplements aids immunity. I recommend both for every child.

AFTERWORD

My patient complains. She saw the doctor upstairs on the fifth floor and he said to put heat on the sore arm. She saw the doctor on the third floor and she said to put cold on it. She saw me on the fourth floor, and I said to leave it alone. Why such a difference and what should the poor patient do?

I understand fully how patients feel in this situation. What I hope with this book is that by learning the principles of why certain therapies work and why placebos work, you will be in a better position to aid your own healing.

You can be fully assured that taking charge of your health issue and engaging your whole body in the therapy is beneficial. Yes, sometimes putting heat or cold or leaving it alone all work equally well! What does work is using the Whole Body Approach and, probably most important of all, *doing it with a smile.*

Best of health to you.

GLOSSARY

Adenoids. Lymph glands that sit in the upper airway between the nose and the back of the throat that help the body prevent or fight infection by removing bacteria and germs.

Adrenaline. A fight-or-flight hormone produced by the adrenal gland when the body is under stress. Adrenaline inhibits the functioning of disease-fighting white blood cells and suppresses the body's immune defense.

Allergen. A substance that provokes an allergic response.

Allergy. An overreaction of the immune system to a normally harmless substance.

Antibiotics. Drugs that kill bacteria or slow down their reproduction. By doing this, it helps the body's own immune defenders, such as the white blood cells and various antibodies, to clear the bacteria from the body.

Antibiotic resistance. An intense and widespread use of antibiotics, not only for sinusitis but also for ear infections, respiratory tract infections, and more, has led to a serious global problem, which is bacterial resistance to common antibiotics.

Antibody. An immune-system protein that is designed to intercept and neutralize a specific invading organisms or other foreign substance; the chief antibody of the allergic reaction is immunoglobulin E (*see* IgE).

Antigen. Any substance (for example, pollen) that provokes an allergic response.

Antihistamines. Over-the-counter and prescription medicines that interfere with the action of histamines by attaching to histamine receptors on cells (*see* histamine).

Atopy. A genetic predisposition toward allergy.

Biofilm. A protective coating that develops around bacteria that can keep antibiotics and white blood cell defenders from getting at it.

CT scan. A computed tomography scan. A computerized x-ray technique used to create a three-dimensional image for the purpose of detecting abnormalities; a CT scan is the best method for viewing the sinuses.

Corticosteroids. A type of anti-inflammatory medicine often referred to by the shortened term "steroids."

Cortisol. A fight-or-flight hormone produced by the adrenal gland when the body is under stress. Cortisol inhibits the functioning of disease-fighting white blood cells and suppresses the body's immune defense.

Decongestant. Drugs that help reduce nasal congestion.

Eosinophils. A type of white blood cell associated with allergic reactions.

Guaifenesin. An expectorant used to help clear mucus from the chest. It works by thinning the mucus in the lungs. It is available both over-the-counter (Mucinex, Robitussin, and others) and by prescription and in tablet, capsule, and liquid forms.

Histamine. A chemical released by the immune system that dilates blood vessels and sets off allergic symptoms.

Immune system. Cells and proteins that work to protect the body from harmful, infectious microorganisms such as bacteria, viruses, and fungi.

Immunity. The ability of the body to resist and overcome infection and disease.

Immunoglobulin. A protein that functions as an antibody in the body's immune response; immunoglobulins are made by white blood cells and are found in body fluids and mucous membranes (*see* Antibody).

Immunoglobulin E (IgE). A type of antibody produced by the immune system when an allergen enters the body. Atopic individuals have a genetic predisposition to make exaggerated amounts of this protective protein.

Larynx. Voice box. The larynx is situated at the crossroads of the air and food passages.

Leukotriene. A powerful immune chemical that, in excess, produces a battery of damaging chemicals that can cause inflammation and spasms in the airways of people with asthma.

Lysozyme. An enzyme found in nasal secretions and many other body fluids that dissolves bacteria.

Magnestic resonance imaging (MRI). An imaging technique that uses radio waves and magnets to view the brain; a functional MRI (fMRI) images the action of glucose in the brain.

Mucous membrane. The soft lining that covers the many cavities and passageways of the body, such as the nasal passages and respiratory tract; the lining produces a clear liquid called mucus.

Nasal septum. The wall dividing the nasal cavity into halves; it is composed of a central supporting skeleton covered on each side by mucous membrane.

Myringotomy. An incision made through the eardrum.

Nodules. Small growths that develop on the vocal cords.

Otolaryngologist. A surgeon who specializes in ear, nose, and throat problems.

Nasal polyps. Small (usually benign) growths in the nasal passage that block mucus drainage and restrict airflow.

Proteolytic enzymes. A group of enzymes that help digest protein as well as thin mucus.

Sinusitis. An inflammation of the nasal sinuses.

Turbinate. A group of shelf-like bony structures that protrude in the nasal passages and help warm and clean the air passing through.

White blood cells. Disease-fighting blood cells that protect the body against dangerous organisms like bacteria, viruses, and fungi, and that are considered its first line of defense.

RESOURCES

SUGGESTED READING

Berger, William. *Allergy and Asthma for Dummies.* Foster City, CA: IDG Books, 2001.

Fenster, Carol. *100 Best Quick Gluten –Free Recipes.* Boston: Houghton Mifflin, 2014.

Grossan Murray. *Stressed? Anxiety? Your Cure Is in the Mirror.* CreateSpace Independent Publishing, 2010.

Grossan Murray. *The Whole Person Tinnitus Relief Program.* Mission Hills, CA: Hydro Med Inc., 2014.

Josephson, Jordan. *Sinus Relief Now.* New York: Perigree Trade, 2006.

Langer, Helen. *A Proven Way to Think Yourself Younger and Healthier.* London: Hodder & Houghton, 2010.

Marks, David and Laura Marks. *The Headache Prevention Cookbook.* New York: Houghton Mifflin Company, 2000.

Martin, Christopher. *Having Nasal Surgery? Don't You Become An Empty Nose Victim!* Nashville, TN: Cold Tree Press, 2007.

Audiovisual Links

Anatomy pictures of the sinuses cavities, nasal passages, and certain disease conditions: www.grossan.com/WBA.sinuspics
Demonstration of office Proetz procedures:
www.youtube.com/watch?v=Nv3gEuPE2_wC
Demonstration of ethmoid implantation:
www.youtube.com/watch?v=lmC-fVwhUOU

Allergy and Sinus Products and Information

In United States

Allergy Buyer's Club
45 Braintree Hill Park, Suite 300
Braintree, MA 02184
(888) 236–7231
www.allergybuyersclub.com

BreathePure Nasal Air Filter
BreathePure Healthcare
P.O. Box 91019
Santa Barbara, CA 93130
(805) 689-7234
http://breathepurenap.com
A popular self-adhering nasal dust/allergy filter.

Hydro Med, Inc.
10200 Sepulveda Blvd.
Mission Hills, CA 91345
(800) 560-9007 or
   (818) 893-6202
www.hydromedonline.com
For questions about Breathe-ease XL Moisturizing Gel, Breathe-ease XL Moisturizing Spray, Breathe-ease XL Nasal Irrigation Solution,

and the Hydro Pulse Nasal and Sinus Irrigation System.

National Allergy Supply
1620 Satellite Blvd. Suite D
Duluth, Georgia 30097
(800) 522-1448

NIOSH-Approved N95
   Filter Mask
These filter masks are available at most pharmacies.

Pasteur Pharmacy
806 Lexington Avenue
New York, NY 10065
(212) 838-2500
maggiekrx@gmail.com
Manhattan source for sinus and allergy products.

Simply Saline Nasal Relief
   Spray
This popular nasal moisturizer contains no preservatives and is available at all pharmacies.

Wellington S. Tichenor, M.D.
642 Park Avenue
New York, NY
(212) 517-6611
www.sinuses.com
For the latest in allergy and sinus news.

In China

Wuhan Ourcare Ltd.
Michael Zhou
Cyberport Dongxing Road
East Lake High-Tech
   Development Zone
Wuhan, People's Republic of
   China
0086 131 6337 3998
www.grossan.taobao.com
www.grossan.cn

SELF-HELP SMELL TESTS

Anosmia Foundation
www.anosmiafoundation.com/
   smelltests.shtml

Sensonics, Inc.
P.O. Box 112
Haddon Heights, NJ 08035
(800) 547-8838
www.sensonics.com/brief-smell-
   landing-page.html

COMPOUNDING PHARMACIES

ASL Pharmacy
900 Calle Plano, Suite M
Camarillo, CA 93012
(866) 552-7579
www.aslrx.com
A source for medications to add to the Hydro-Pulse for sinus irrigation, as well as topical sinus therapies; on prescription, the irrigator is provided with the medication by insurance.

QmedRx
630 North Wymore Road,
   Suite 370
Maitland, FL 32751
(888) 273-9820
www.qmedrx.com
They fill prescription medications to add to the Hydro Pulse for sinus irrigation; on prescription, the irrigator is provided with the medication by insurance.

SUPPORT ORGANIZATIONS

Support groups exist for most illnesses and symptoms, including allergies and sinus-related problems. Start by checking the resources at your local hospital and by doing a search on Google. Facebook has support groups for empty nose syndrome, chronic obstructive pulmonary disorder, and other conditions, where patients themselves may offer their experience and recommendations, but these may not be medical recommendations.

Anosmia Foundation
www.anosmiafoundation.com

American Academy of Allergy,
  Asthma & Immunology
  (AAAAI)
555 East Wells Street,
  Suite 1100
Milwaukee, WI 53202
(414) 272-6071
www.aaaai.org

American Academy of Sleep
  Medicine
2510 North Frontage Road
Darien, IL 60561
(630) 737-9700
www.aasmnet.org

Asthma and Allergy Foundation
  of America (AAFA)
8201 Corporate Drive, Suite 1000
Landover, MD 20785
(800) 727-8462
www.aafa.org

Chronic Obstructive Pulmonary
  Disorder (COPD)
COPD Foundation
20 F Street NW, Suite 200-A
Washington, DC 20001
(866) 731-2673
www.copdfoundation.org

Empty Nose Syndrome:
  A Self-Help Website
EmptyNoseSyndromeOrg
  @gmail.com
www.emptynosesyndrome.org

WHERE TO FIND AN EAR, NOSE, AND THROAT DOCTOR

American Academy of Otolaryngology—
    Head and Neck Surgery
1650 Diagonal Road
Alexandria, VA 22314
(703) 836-4444
www.entnet.org

WHERE TO CONTACT THE AUTHOR

Grossan Sinus and Health Institute
Cedars-Sinai Medical Towers
8631 W. 3rd Street, Suite #440E
Los Angeles, CA 90048
(310) 657-7704
www.grossaninstitute.com
www.towerENT.com

MISCELLANEOUS

The Didgeridoo Store
49522 Road 426
Oakhurst, CA 93644
(866) 468-3434
www.didgeridoostore.com/
    howtoplay.html
Information on where to buy and how to play this ancient wind instrument.

Mosaic Physical Therapy
11835 W. Olympic Blvd
Suite 135E
Los Angeles, CA 90064
310-401-6410
www.mosaicpt.com
Provides information on the physiology of why physical therapy works for headaches and sinus pain.

REFERENCES

Introduction

Marek RJ, AR Block, YS Ben-Porath. "The Minnesota Multiphasic Personality Inventory-2-Restructured Form (MMPI-2-RF): Incremental Validity in Predicting Early Postoperative Outcomes in Spine Surgery Candidates." *Psychol Assess* 2014 [Epub ahead of print].

Tavernise S. "U.S. Aims to Curb Peril of Antibiotic Resistance." *New York Times,* Sept 19, 2014, A16.

Chapter 1: The Whole Body Approach

Allen D. "Laughter Really Can Be the Best Medicine." *Nurs Stand* 2014; 28(32): 24–25.

Centers for Disease Control and Prevention. *MMWR Morb Mortal Wkly Rep* 2013 Jan 4; 61(51–52): 1033–1037.

Cohen S. "Positive Emotional Style Predicts Resistance to Illness after Experimental Exposure to Rhinovirus or Influenza A Virus." *Psychosom Med* 2006; 68: 809–815.

Cohen S. "Psychological Stress and Susceptibility to the Common Cold." *N Engl J Med* 1991; 325: 606–612.

Cousins N. *Anatomy of an Illness as Perceived by the Patient: Reflections on Healing.* New York: W.W. Norton & Co, 1979.

Crum AJ, EJ Langer. "Mind-Set Matters: Exercise and the Placebo Effect." *Psychol Sci* 2007; 18(2): 165–171.

Grossan M. "A Brief Introduction to Biofeedback for Otolaryngologists." *ORL Digest* 1975; 37: 15–19.

Hassed C. "Mind-Body Therapies-Use in Chronic Pain Management." *Aust Fam Physician* 2013; 42(3): 112–117.

Hens G, PW Hellings. "The Nose: Gatekeeper and Trigger of Bronchial Disease." *Rhinology.* 2006; 44(3): 179–187.

Krämer U, R Schmitz, J Ring, et al. "What Can Reunification of East and West Germany Tell Us About the Cause of the Allergy Epidemic?" *Clin Exp Allergy.* 2014 Nov 21. [Epub ahead of print]

Langer E, M Djikic, M Pirson, et al. "Believing Is Seeing: Using Mindlessness (Mindfully) to Improve Visual Acuity." *Psychol Sci* 2010; 21(5): 661–666.

Langer E. *Counterclockwise: Mindful Health and the Power of Possibility.* New York: Ballentine, 2009.

Mallett J. "Humor and Laughter Therapy." *Complement Ther Nurs Midwifery* 1995; 1(3): 73–76.

van Buchem FL, JA Knottnerus, VJ Schrijnemaekers, et al. "Primary-Care-Based Randomised Placebo-Controlled Trial of Antibiotic Treatment in Acute Maxillary Sinusitis." *Lancet* 1997; 349: 683–687.

Wild B. "Neural Correlated of Laughter and Humor." *Brain* 2003; 126: 2121–2138.

Chapter 2: What Is Allergy and Why Did I Get It?

Baroody FM, RM Naclerio. "Immunology of the Upper Airway and Pathophysiology and Treatment of Allergic Rhinitis." In *Cummings Otolaryngology: Head & Neck*

Surgery edited by PW Flint, et al. 5th ed. China: Mosby Elsevier, 2010.

Berg O. "Occurrence of Asymptomatic Sinusitis in Common Cold and Other Acute ENT-Infections." *Rhinology* 1986; 24: 223.

Braunstahl GJ. "United Airways Concept: What Does It Teach Us about Systemic Inflammation in Airways Disease?" *Proc Am Thorac* Soc 2009; 6(8): 652–654.

Brooks C, N Pearce, J Douwes. The Hygiene Hypothesis in Allergy and Asthma: An Update. *Curr Opin Allergy Clin Immunol* 2013; 13: 70–77.

Gould H et al. "The Biology of IgE and the Basis of Allergic Disease." *Annu Rev Immunol* 2003; 21: 579–628.

Grossan M. "The Saccharin Test of Nasal Mucociliary Function." *The Eye Ear Nose and Throat Monthly* 1975; 54: 415–417.

Lee JK, P Vadas. "Anaphylaxis: Mechanisms and Management." *Clin Exp Allergy* 2011; 41(7): 923–938.

Meltzer EO, J Szwarcberg, MW Pill. "Allergic Rhinitis, Asthma, and Rhinosinusitis: Diseases of the Integrated Airway." *J Manag Care Pharm* 2004; 10(4): 310–317.

Proetz AW. "Air Currents in the Upper Respiratory Tract and Their Clinical Importance." *Ann Oto Rhin Laryn* 1951; 60: 439–467.

Strachan DB. Hay fever, hygiene, and household size. *BMJ* 1989; 299: 1259–1260.

Subiza JL, J Subiza, MC Barjau. "Inhibition of the Seasonal IgE Increases to Dactylis glomerata by Daily Sodium Nasal-Sinus Irrigation During the Grass Pollen Season." *J Allergy Clin Immunol* 1999; 104(3): 711–712.

Von Hertzen LC, T Haahtela. "Asthma and Atopy: The Price of Affluence?" *Allergy* 2004; 59(2): 124–137.

Chapter 3: What Works for Allergy and Why?

Benedetti F, HS Mayberg, TD Wager TD, et al. "Neurobiological Mechanisms of the Placebo Effect." *J Neurosci* 2005; 25(45): 10390–10402.

Grossan M. *Free Yourself from Sinus and Allergy Problems—Permanently.* Mission Hills, CA: Hydro Med, 2009.

Grossan M. *Stressed? Anxiety? Your Cure is in the Mirror.* Mission Hills, CA: Hydro Med, 2012.

Jacobson E. *Modern Treatment of Tense Patients.* Springfield, IL: Charles C. Thomas, 1970.

Johns Hopkins Med Lett Health After 50. "Why Are Placebos Important in Clinical Trials, and Why Do They Sometimes 'Work'?" 2006; 18(9): 8.

Laekeman G, S Simoens, J Buffels. "Continuous versus On-Demand Pharmacotherapy of Allergic Rhinitis: Evidence and Practice." *Respir Med* 2010; 104(5): 615–625.

Marglani O. Update in the Management of Allergic Fungal Sinusitis." *Saudi Med J* 2014; 35(8): 791–795.

Okereke OI, J Prescott, YY Jason, et al. "High Phobic Anxiety Is Related to Lower Leukocyte Telomere Length in Women." *PLoS One* 2012; 7(7): e40516.

Serrano E, U Wahn H, A Didier, et al. "300IR 5-Grass Pollen Sublingual Tablet Offers Relief from Nasal Symptoms in Patients with Allergic Rhinitis." *Am J Rhinol Allergy* 2014 Oct 20. [Epub ahead of print]

Wilson MT, DL Hamilos. "The Nasal and Sinus Microbiome in Health and Disease. *Curr Allergy Asthma Rep* 2014; 14(12): 485.

Chapter 4: Why Did I Get Sinusitis?

Boek WM, N Keles, K Graamans, et al. "Physiologic and Hypertonic Saline Solutions Impair Ciliary Activity In Vitro." *Laryngoscope* 1999; 109(3): 396–399.

Folker RJ, BF Marple, RL Mabry. "Treatment of Allergic Fungal Sinusitis: A Comparison Trial of Postoperative Immunotherapy with Specific Fungal Antigens." *Laryngoscope* 1998; 108: 1623–1627.

Fontanari P, H Burnet, MC Zattara-Hartmann, et al. "Changes in Airway Resistance Induced by Nasal Inhalation of Cold Dry, Dry, or Moist Air in Normal Individuals." *J Appl Physiol* 1996; 81(4): 1739–1743.

Grossan M. "The Saccharin Test of Nasal Mucociliary Function." *The Eye Ear Nose and Throat Monthly* 1975; 54(11): 415–417.

Hens G, PW Hellings. "The Nose: The Gatekeeper and Trigger of Bronchial Disease." *Rhinology* 2006; 44: 179–187.

Houser SM, KJ Keen. "The Role of Allergy and Smoking in Chronic Rhinosinusitis and Polyposis." *Laryngoscope* 2008; 118(9): 1521–1527.

Li L, D Han, L Zhang, et al. Aerodynamic Investigation of the Correlation Between Nasal Septal Deviation and Chronic Rhinosinusitis." *Laryngoscope* 2012; 122(9): 1915–1919.

Manning SC, RL Mabry, SD Schaefer, et al. "Evidence of IgE-Mediated Hypersensitivity in Allergic Fungal Sinusitis." *Laryngoscope* 1993; 103(7): 717–721.

Ramadan HH, AD Meyers, LG Close, et al. "Fungal Sinusitis." Medscape, accessed Jan 15 2012, http://emedicine.medscape.com/article/863062-overview.

Snow SJ, J McGee, DB Miller, et al. "Inhaled Diesel Emissions Generated with Cerium Oxide Nanoparticle Fuel Additive Induce Adverse Pulmonary and Systemic Effects." *Toxicol Sci* 2014. [Epub ahead of print]

Wellington S, WS Tichenor, J Thurlow. "Nontuberculous mycobacteria in household plumbing as possible cause of chronic rhinosinusitis." *Emerg Infect Diseases* 2012; 18(10): 1612–1617.

Yang SN, CC Hsieh, HF Kuo, et al. "The Effects of Environmental Toxins on Allergic Inflammation." *Allergy Asthma Immunol Res* 2014; 6(6):478–484.

Chapter 5: What to Do for Your Sinusitis

Benninger MS. "The Pathogenesis of Rhinosinusitis." In *Cummings Otolaryngology: Head & Neck Surgery* edited by PW Flint, et al. 5th ed. China: Mosby Elsevier, 2010.

Bucher HC, P Tschudi, J Young, et al. "Effect of Amoxicillin-Clavulanate in Clinically Diagnosed Acute Rhinosinusitis: A Placebo-Controlled, Double-Blind, Randomized Trial in General Practice." *Arch Intern Med* 2003; 163(15): 1793–1798.

Jervis-Bardy J, S Boase, A Psalti, et al. "A Randomized Trial of Mupirocin Sinonasal Rinses Versus Saline in Surgically Recalcitrant Staphylococcal Chronic Rhinosinusitis." *Laryngoscope* 2012; 122(10): 2148–2152.

Keen M. "The Clinical Significance of Nasal Irrigation Bottle Contamination." *Laryngoscope* 2010: 120(10): 2110–2014.

Lee JM, Nayak JV, Doghramji LL. "Assessing the Risk of Irrigation Bottle and Fluid Contamination." *Am J Rhinol Allergy* 2010; 24(3): 197–199.

Macri GF, A Greco. Evidence and Role of Autoantibodies in Chronic Rhinosinusitis with Nasal Polyps." *Int J Immunopathol Pharmacol* 2014; 27(2): 155–161.

Nsouli T. "Long-Term Use of Nasal Saline Irrigation: Harmful or Helpful?" Paper presented at the American College of Allergy, Asthma & Immunology Annual Meeting, Washington, DC, Nov 8, 2009.

Proença M, F Pitta, D Kovelis, et al. D "Mucociliary Clearance and Its Relation with the Level of Physical Activity in Daily Life In Healthy Smokers and Nonsmokers." *Rev Port Pneumol* 2012 18(5): 233–238.

Sakallio?lu Ö, IA Güvenç, C Cingi. "Xylitol and Its Usage in ENT Practice. *J Laryngol Otol* 2014; 128(7): 580–585.

Chapter 6: Is It a Cold, a Sinus Infection, or an Allergy?

Cohen S, WJ Doyle, CM Alper, et al. "Sleep Habits and Susceptibility to the Common Cold." *Arch Intern Med* 2009; 169(1): 62–67.

Costa ML, AJ Psaltis, JV Nayak, et al. "Long-Term Outcomes of Endoscopic Maxillary Mega-Antrostomy for Refractory Chronic Maxillary Sinusitis." *Int Forum Allergy Rhinol* 2014 Oct 13. [Epub ahead of print]

Das RR, Singh M. "Oral Zinc for e Common Cold." *JAMA* 2014; 311(14):1440–1441.

Houser SM, HL Levine. "Chronic Daily Headache: When to Suspect Sinus Disease." *Curr Pain Headache Rep* 2008; 12(1): 45–49.

Karsch-Völk M, B Barrett B, D Kiefer, et al. "Echinacea for Preventing and Treating the Common Cold." *Cochrane Database Syst Rev* 2014, doi: 10.1002/14651858 .CD000530 .pub3.

Simasek M, DA Blandino. "Treatment of the Common Cold." *Am Fam Physician* 2007; 75(4): 515–520.

Chapter 7: Is It a Sinus Headache, a Tension Headache, or a Migraine?

Bartleson JD, FM Cutrer. "Migraine Update: Diagnosis and Treatment." *Minn Med* 2010; 93(5): 36–41.

Centers for Disease Control and Prevention. "Sleep and Sleep Disorders." July 2013. Available at: www.cdc.gov/sleep.

Cevoli S, G Giannini, V Favoni, et al. "Migraine and Sleep Disorders." *Neurol Sci* 2012; 33 Suppl 1: S43–46.

Crane J, DI Ogborn, C Cupido. "Massage Therapy Attenuates Inflammatory Signaling After Exercise-Induced Muscle Damage." *Sci Transl Med* 2012; 4(119): 119ra13.

Goldstein J, Hagen M, Gold M. "Results of a Multicenter, Double-Blind, Randomized, Parallel-Group, Placebo-Controlled, Single-Dose Study Comparing the Fixed Combination of Acetaminophen, Acetylsalicylic Acid, and Caffeine with Ibuprofen for Acute Treatment of Patients with Severe Migraine." *Cephalalgia* 2014; 34(13): 1070-1078.

Grossan, M. "Treatment of Migraine with a Vasodilator-Nicotinyl Alcohol." *ORL Digest* 1975; 86(6): 936–937.

Grossan M. "Treatment of Temporomandibular Joint Disease with Biofeedback." In: *The Temporomandibular Joint: A Biological Basis for Clinical Practice* edited by Leland House. Philadelphia, PA: WB Saunders Co., 1989.

Headache Classification Subcommittee of the International Headache Society. "The International Classification of Headache Disorders." 2nd ed. *Cephalalgia* 2004; 24 (Suppl 1): 9–160.

Houser SM, HL Levine. "Chronic Daily Headache: When to Suspect Sinus Disease."

Current Pain and Headache Reports 2008; 12(1): 45–49.

Lal D, A Rounds, DW Dodick. "Comprehensive Management of Patients Presenting to the Otolaryngologist for Sinus Pressure, Pain, or Headache." *Laryngoscope.* 2014 Sep 12. [Epub ahead of print]

Nestoriuc Y, A Martin, W Rief, et al. "Biofeedback Treatment for Headache Disorders: A Comprehensive Efficacy Review." *AAPB* 2008; 33(3): 125–140.

Nestoriuc Y, M Alexandra. "Efficacy of Biofeedback for Migraine: A Meta-Analysis." *Pain* 2007; 128(1–2): 111–127.

Olesen J, P Tfelt-Hansen, K Michael, et al. *The Headaches.* 3rd ed. Philadelphia, PA: Lippincott Williams & Wilkins, 2006.

Reed KL, SB Black, CJ Banta, et al. "Combined Occipital and Supraorbital Neurostimulation for the Treatment of Chronic Migraine Headaches: Initial Experience." *Cephalalgia* 2010; 30(3): 260–271.

Rockett FC, VR de Oliveira, K Castro, et al. "Dietary Aspects of Migraine Trigger Factors." *Nutr Rev* 2012 Jun; 70(6): 337–356.

Roozbahany NA, S Nasri. "Nasal and Paranasal Sinus Anatomical Variations in Patients with Rhinogenic Contact Point Headache." *Auris Nasus Larynx* 2013; 40(2): 177–183.

Sleep Disorders and Sleep Deprivation: An Unmet Public Health Problem edited by Harvey Colton and Bruce Altevogt. Washington, DC: The National Academies Press, 2006.

Wahabi HA, LA Alansary, AH Al-Sabban, et al. "The Effectiveness of *Hibiscus sabdariffa* in the Treatment of Hypertension: A Systematic Review." *Phytomedicine* 2010; 17(2): 83–86.

Chapter 8: How to Clear Postnasal Drip and Thick Mucus

Alvar A. "Prevention of Exacerbations in Chronic Obstructive Pulmonary Disease: Knowns and Unknowns." *J COPD Foundation* 2014 1(2): 166-184.

Boek WM, N Keles, K Graamans K. "Physiologic and Hypertonic Saline Solutions Impair Ciliary Activity in Vitro." *Laryngoscope* 1999; 109(3): 396–399.

Braido F, I Baiardini, D Lacedonia, et al. "Sleep Apnea Risk in Patients with Asthma with or without Comorbid Rhinitis." *Respir Care* 2014. [Epub ahead of print]

Grossan M. "Enhancing the Mucociliary System." *Advance for Respiratory Care Practitioners.* 1995; 8: 12–13.

Grossan M. "Nasal Function: Office Measurement of Nasal Mucociliary Clearance." In *Otolaryngology* Vol 2. Philadelphia: Lippincott Williams & Wilkins, 1994.

Hellgren J, AC Olin, K Torén. "Increased Risk of Rhinitis Symptoms in Subjects with Gastroesophageal Reflux." *Acta Otolaryngol* 2014; 134(6): 615–619.

Nsouli TM. "Long-Term Use of Nasal Saline Irrigation: Harmful or Helpful?" Abstract #32: Oral presentation at the ACAAI Annual Meeting, Washington, DC, November 8, 2009.

Rosenberg M. "Clinical Assessment of Bad Breath: Current Concepts." *J Am Dent Assoc* 1996; 127(4): 475–482.

Weber CS. "Common Infections of the Ear, Nose, and Throat." *Kleinjung T. Praxis* 2014; 103(17): 1001–1007.

Chapter 9: How the Sinuses Affect Asthma and Other Lung Conditions

American Lung Association. "Chronic Obstructive Pulmonary Disease (COPD) Fact Sheet." May 2014. Available at: www.lung.org/lung-disease/copd/resources/facts-figures/COPD-Fact-Sheet.html.

Benninger MS, CE Holy. "The Impact of Endoscopic Sinus Surgery on Health Care Use in Patients with Respiratory Comorbidities." *Otolaryngol Head Neck Surg* 2014; 151(3): 508–515.

Chakravorty I, K Chahal, G Austin. "A Pilot Study of the Impact of High-Frequency Chest Wall Oscillation in Chronic Obstructive Pulmonary Disease Patients with Mucus Hypersecretion." *Int J Chron Obstruct Pulmon Dis* 2011; 6: 693–699.

Centers for Disease Control and Prevention. National Center for Health Statistics. *National Vital Statistics Reports* 2013; 61(4), May 8, 2013.

Centers for Disease Control and Prevention. "Sleep and Sleep Disorders." July 2013. Available at: www.cdc.gov/sleep.

Decramer M. "Treatment of COPD: The Sooner the Better." *Thorax* 2010; 65(9): 837–841.

Fontanari P, MC Zattara-Hartmann, H Burnet, et al. "Nasal Eupnoeic Inhalation of Cold, Dry Air Increases Airway Resistance in Asthmatic Patients." *Eur Respir J* 1997; 10(10): 2250–2254.

Hens G, BM Vanaudenaerde, DM Bullens, et al. "Sinonasal Pathology in Nonallergic Asthma and COPD: 'United Airway Disease' beyond the Scope of Allergy." *Allergy* 2008; 63(3): 261–267.

Laniado-Laborín R. "Smoking and Chronic Obstructive Pulmonary Disease (COPD)." *Int J Environ Res Public Health* 2009; 6(1): 209–224.

Mahler DA. "Mechanisms and Measurement of Dyspnea in Chronic Obstructive Pulmonary Disease." *PATS* 2006; 3(3): 234–238.

Mason, RJ, VC Broaddus, JF Murray, et al. "Asthma." In *Murray and Nadel's Textbook of Respiratory Medicine* edited by RJ Mason, et al. 4th ed. Philadelphia: Elsevier Saunders, 2005.

Marcinuk D. "Optimizing Pulmonary Rehabilitation in Chronic Obstructive Pulmonary Disease." *Can Resp Jour* 2010; 17(4): 159–168.

Miravitles M. "Chronic Obstructive Pulmonary Disease." *Lancet* 2012; 379: 1341–1351.

Murphy KR, EO Meltzer, MS Blaiss, et al. "Asthma Management and Control in the United States: Results of the 2009 Asthma Insight And Management Survey." *Allergy Asthma Proc* 2012; 33(1): 54–64.

O'Donnell DE. "Hyperinflation, Dyspnea, and Exercise Intolerance in Chronic Obstructive Pulmonary Disease." *PATS* 2006; 3(2): 180–184.

Ozagar A, F Dede, T Turoglu, et al. "Aspiration of Nasal Secretions the Lungs of Patients with Acute Sinonasal Infections." *Laryngoscope* 2000; 110(1): 107–110.

Pinto JM, KE Wroblewski, DW Kern, et al. "Olfactory Dysfunction Predictis 5-Year Mortality in Older Adults." *PLoS One* 2014, doi: 10,1371/journal.pone.0107541.

Sleep Disorders and Sleep Deprivation: An Unmet Public Health Problem edited by Harvey Colton and Bruce Altevogt. Washington, DC: The National Academies Press, 2006.

Spruit MA. American Thoracic Society Advances in Pulmonary Rehabilitation. *Am J Respir Care Med* 2013; 188(8): e13–64.

Von Hertzen LC, T Haahtela. "Asthma and Atopy: The Price of Affluence?" *Allergy* 2004; 59(2): 124–137.

Chapter 10: How to Treat Throat and Voice Problems

Cammarota G, G Masala, R Cianci, et al. "Reflux Symptoms in Professional Opera Choristers." *Gastroenterology* 2007; 132(3): 890–898.

Gonsalves A, E Amin, M Behlau. "Overall Voice and Strain Level Analysis in Rock Singers." *Pro Fono* 2010; 22(3): 195–200.

Sataloff RT. "Professional Voice Users: The Evaluation of Voice Disorders." *Occup Med* 2001; 16(4): 633–647.

Chapter 11: How to Stop Snoring without Surgery

Almeida FR, N Henrich, C Marra. "Patient Preferences and Experiences of CPAP and Oral Appliances for the Treatment of Obstructive Sleep Apnea: A Qualitative Analysis." *Sleep Breath* 2013; 17(2): 659–666.

American Academy of Sleep Medicine. Practice Guidelines. 2014. Available at: www .aasmnet.org/Resources/clinicalguidelines/OSA.

Kim YK, Hong SL, Yoon EJ, Kim SE, Kim JW. "Central Presentation of Postviral Olfactory Loss Evaluated By Positron Emission Tomography Scan: A Pilot Study." *Am J Rhinol Allergy* 2012; 26(3): 204–208.

Koinis-Mitchell D, T Craig, CA Esteban, et al. "Sleep and Allergic Disease: A summary of the Literature and Future Directions for Research." *J Allergy Clin Immunol* 2012; 130: 1275–1281.

Lim DJ, SH Kang, BH Kim, et al. "Treatment of Obstructive Sleep Apnea Syndrome Using Radiofrequency-Assisted Uvulopalatoplasty with Tonsillectomy." *Eur Arch Otorhinolaryngol* 2013; 270(2): 585–593.

Nieto FJ, PE Peppard, T Young, et al. "Sleep-Disordered Breathing and Cancer Mortality: Results from the Wisconsin Sleep Cohort Study." *Am J Respir Crit Care Med* 2012; 186(2): 190–194.

Chapter 13: How to Limit the Health Effects of Smog, Fires, and Volcano Gases

Analitis A, I Georgiadis, K Katsouyanni. "Forest Fires Are Associated with Elevated Mortality in a Dense Urban Setting." *Occup Environ Med* 2012; 69(3): 158–162.

Armentia A, T Asensio, J Subiza, et al. "Living in Towers as Risk Factor of Pollen Allergy." *Allergy* 2004; 59(3): 302–305.

Bernstein AS, SS Myers. "Climate Change and Children's Health." *Curr Opin Pediatr* 2011; 23(2): 221–226.

Johnson DB, N Oyama, L LeMarchand, et al. "Native Hawaiians Mortality, Morbidity, and Lifestyle: Comparing Data from 1982, 1990, and 2000." *Pac Health Dialog* 2004; 11(2): 120–130.

Likcso D, TL Guidotti, DE Franklin, et al. "Indoor Environmental and Air Quality Characteristics, Building-Related Health Symptoms, and Worker Productivity in a Federal Government Building Complex." *Arch Environ Occup Health* 2014 Sept 25. [Epub ahead of print]

Wegesser TC, KE Pinkerton, JA Last. "California Wildfires of 2008: Coarse and Fine Particulate Matter Toxicity." *Environ Health Perspect* 2009; 117(6): 893–897.

Weinhold B. "Fields and Forests in Flames: Vegetation Smoke & Human Health." *Environ Health Perspect* 2011; 119(9): a386–393.

Chapter 14: How to Resolve Other Nasal- and Sinus-Related Conditions

Bachert C, P Gevaert, P van Cauwenberge. "Nasal Polyps and Rhinosinusitis." In: *Middleton's Allergy: Principles and Practice* edited by NF Adkinson, et al. 7th ed. Philadelphia, PA: Mosby Elsevier, 2008.

Chhabra N, Houser SM. "The Diagnosis and Management of Empty Nose Syndrome." *Otolaryngol Clin North Am* 2009; 42(2): 311–30, ix.

Houser SM. "Surgical Treatment for Empty Nose Syndrome." *Arch Otolaryngol Head Neck Surg* 2007; 133(9): 858–863.

Houser SM. "Empty Nose Syndrome Associated with Middle Turbinate Resection." *Otolaryngol Head Neck Surg* 2006; 135(6): 972–973.

Houser SM. "Does the Method of Inferior Turbinate Surgery Affect the Development of Empty Nose Syndrome?" In *Having Nasal Surgery? Don't You Become An Empty Nose Victim!* by Christopher Martin. Nashville, TN: Cold Tree Press, 2007.

Moore EJ, EB Kern. "Atrophic Rhinitis: A Review of 242 Cases." *Am J Rhinol* 2001; 15(6): 355–361.

Scheithauer MO. "Surgery of the Turbinates and Empty Nose Syndrome." *Curr Top Otorhinolaryngol Head Neck Surg* 2010; 9: 1–28.

Scully C. "Halitosis." *Clin Evid* (Online). 2014 Sep 18. [Epub ahead of print]

Zhang X, F Li , L Zhang, et al. "A Longitu-dinal Study of Sick Building Syndrome (SBS) among Pupils in Relation to SO2, NO2, O3 and PM10 in Schools in China." *PLoS One* 2014; 14; 9(11): e112933.

Chapter 15: When Surgery Is an Option

Chhabra N, Houser SM. "Empty Nose Syndrome: Diagnosis and Management," *Otolaryngol Clin N Am* 2008; 42: 311–330.

Chhabra N, Houser SM. "Endonasal Repair of Septal Perforations Using a Rotational Mucosal Flap." *Int Forum Allergy Rhinol* 2012; 2(5): 392–396.

Grossan M. "Mirror Technique of Nasopharyngeal Surgery." *Ear Nose and Throat Monthly* 1972; 51: 302–305.

Houser SM. "Empty Nose Syndrome Associated with Middle Turbinate Resection," *Otolaryngol HeadNeck Surg* 2006; 135(6): 972–973.

Kern RC, DI Kutler, KJ Reid, et al. "Laser-Assisted Uvulopalatoplasty and Tonsillectomy for the Management of Obstructive Sleep Apnea Syndrome." *Laryngoscope* 2003; 113(7): 1175–1181.

Kim E, JL Cutler. "Balloon Dilatation of the Paranasal Sinuses: A Tool in Sinus Surgery." *Otolaryngol Clin North Am* 2009; 42(5): 847–856.

Lal D, JA Stankiewicz. "Primary Sinus Surgery." In *Cummings Otolaryngology: Head & Neck Surgery* edited by PW Flint, et al. 5th ed. China: Mosby Elsevier, 2010.

Martin C. *Having Nasal Surgery? Don't You Become an Empty Nose Victim.* Nashville, TN: Cold Tree Press, 2007.

Naraghi M, B Amirzargar, A Meysamie. "Quality of Life Comparison in Common

Rhinologic Surgeries." *Allergy Rhinol (Providence)* 2012; 3(1) :1–7.

Ramadan HH, H Bueller, ST Hester, et al. "Sinus Balloon Catheter Dilation after Adenoidectomy Failure for Children with Chronic Rhinosinusitis." *Arch Otolaryngol Head Neck Surg* 2012; 138(7): 635–637.

Sozansky J, S Houser. "Pathophysiology of Empty Nose Syndrome." *Laryngoscope* 2014 Jun 30. [Epub ahead of press]

Weiss RL, CA Church, et al. "Long-Term Outcome Analysis of Balloon Catheter Sinusotomy: Two-Year Follow Up." *Otolaryngol Head Neck Surg* 2008; 139: S38–S46.

Chapter 16: Kid Stuff

Chirco G. "Nasal Congestion in Infancy and Children: A Literature Review on Efficacy and Safety of Non-Pharacological Treatments." *Minerva Pediatr* 2014; 66(6): 549–557.

Grossan M. "The Ins and Outs of Common Ear Problems." *Patient Care* 2002: 56–71.

Grossan M. "Irrigation of the Child's Nose." *Clin Ped* 1974; 13: 229–231.

Grossan M. "Irrigation Treatment for Throat Infections. *Ear Nose and Throat Monthly* 1972; 51: 302–305.

Higuchi O et al. "Relationship between Rhinitis and Nocturnal Cough in School Children." *Pediatr Allergy Immunol* 2012; 23(6): 562–566.

Ioan I, M Poussel, L Coutier. "What Is Chronic Cough in Children?" *Front Physiol* 2014; 28; 5: 322.

Magit A. "Pediatric Rhinosinusitis." *Otolaryngol Clin North Am* 2014; 47(5): 733–746.

Kassel JC, D King, GK Spurling. "Saline Nasal Irrigation for Acute Upper Respiratory Tract Infections." *Cochrane Database Syst Rev* 2010;(3): CD006821.

Liu AH, RA Covar, JD Spahn, et al. "Childhood Asthma." In *Nelson Textbook of Pediatrics* edited by RM Kliegman, et al. 19th ed. Philadelphia, PA: Saunders Elsevier, 2011.

Megan L. "Sleep Disordered Breathing after Adenotonsilectomy." *Arch of Otol* 2012; 138(7): 638–643.

Oduwole O, MM Meremikwu, A Oyo-Ita, et al. "Honey for Acute Cough in Children." *Cochrane Database Syst Rev* 2012; 3: CD007094.

Ownby DR, CC Johnson, EL Peterson. "Exposure to Dogs and Cats in the First Year of Life and Risk of Allergic Sensitization at 6 to 7 Years of Age." *JAMA* 2002; 288(8): 963–972.

Papadopoulou A, D Tsoukala, K Tsoumakas. "Rhinitis and Asthma in Children: Comorbitity or United Airway Disease?" *Curr Pediatr Rev* 2014 Nov 14. [Epub ahead of print]

Perzanowski MS, E Ronmark, TA Platts-Mills, et al. "Effect of Cat and Dog Ownership on Sensitization and Development of Asthma Among Pre-Teenage Children." *Am J Respir Crit Care Med* 2002; 166(5): 696–702.

Piessens P, G Hens, N Lemkens, et al. "Effect of Adenotonsillectomy on the Use of Respiratory Medication." *Int J Pediatr Otorhinolaryngol* 2012; 76(6): 906–910.

Shaikh N, ER Wald, M Pi. "Decongestants, Antihistamines and Nasal Irrigation for Acute Sinusitis in Children." *Cochrane Database Syst Rev.* 2010; 12: CD007909.

INDEX

Accolate, 141
Acid reflux. *See*
  Gastroesophageal
  reflux disease (GERD).
Adenoid facies, 218
Adenoidectomy, 218, 220
Adenoids, 217
  enlarged, 165–166, 192,
  214, 217–218, 219,
  223
Advair Diskus, 140
Affirmations, 152
Afrin, 38, 44, 198, 199,
  200
Afrinol, 44
Air
  cold, 138
  moisturized, 121, 171,
  194, 195
Albuterol, 189
Alcohol, 111
Alexander, Frederick
  Matthias, 157
Alexander Technique, 157
Allegra, 44
Allergens, 23, 25, 26, 28
  indoor, 48–50
  outdoor, 47–48
Allergies, 21–58, 77, 136,
  180, 211
  arithmetic equation of,
  22, 28, 29, 31–32

cat, 32, 36
causes, 23–34
children and, 32
desensitization for, 22,
  28, 43, 65
diagnosing, 34–37
dust, 28–29, 36, 48
environment and, 23–24
food, 22, 25, 32–33,
  36–37, 111, 133–134,
  158, 214, 222
genetics and, 23, 24
medications, 33–34
mold, 29–30, 36, 48,
  49–50
nasal, 21, 25
perennial, 25, 29, 36
pollens, 25, 26–28, 34,
  36, 47
seasonal, 25, 28, 34–36
symptoms, 21, 26,
  31–32, 36, 88–89
tests (blood), 28, 32, 35,
  36
tests (skin), 35
treatment, 40–58, 122
trees, 27, 35
Allergy drops. *See* Sub-
  lingual immunization
  therapy (SLIT).
Allergy shots. *See* Injections,
  desensitization.

AlloDerm, 208
Alupent, 140
Alveoli, 136, 147
Alzheimer's disease, 178
Amerge, 107
American Academy of
  Allergy, Asthma, and
  Immunology, 49
American Academy of
  Neurology, 107
American Academy of
  Sleep Medicine, 172,
  173
American Headache
  Society, 107
Ammonia, 69
Amphotericin B, 65
Amygdala, 12
Anaphylaxis, 22
Anosmia. *See* Smell, loss of.
Anosmia Foundation, 179
Antibiotics, 3, 10–11, 64,
  65, 75–76, 85–87, 97,
  199
  side effects, 80
Antibodies. *See*
  Immunoglobulins (Ig).
Anticholinergics, 141, 149
Antigens, 22–23
Antihistamines, 41, 44,
  122, 130, 195
Anxiety, 13, 94, 142

Anxiety reinforcement, 11,
    13–14
Apnea episodes, 167
Ariflo, 150
Aspirin, 143, 195, 212
Astelin, 38, 44
Astepro, 44, 122, 130
Asthma, 25, 30, 41, 57,
    59, 64, 136–146, 159
    measuring, 138–139
    medication instructions
        and, 142, 145–146
    medications, 140–142
    symptoms, 137
    triggers, 138, 142–143,
        144
    undiagnosed, 139–140
    whole body approach
        (WBA) to, 140–146
Atopy, 23, 24, 32, 136
Atrovent, 38, 141, 149
Atrovent HFA, 141
Auras, 106
Avoidance, 47–50, 222
Ayr Gel, 196

Bacon, 112
Bacteria, 84, 86, 97, 126,
    128
    intestinal, 64, 66, 84
Bactroban, 191, 195, 197,
    208
Bae, Charles, 172
Bananas, 195
Barrel chests, 147
Bathrooms, 49
Beans, 112
Beconase, 44
Bedrooms, 48, 49, 72,
    171, 194, 195, 214
Beds, 146
Benadryl, 44, 94, 122, 199
Benzalkonium, 198

Benzedrex, 104, 122
Bernoulli effect, 82, 86
Beta2-adrenergic agonists,
    140
    side effects, 141
Beta2-agonists. See Beta2-
    adrenergic agonists.
Biaxin, 211
Bifocals, 118
Biofeedback, 13, 50,
    78–79, 117, 152, 159,
    193
Biofilm, 76, 86, 128
Bioflavonoids, 195
Biotine Oral Rinse, 130
Birth control pills, 115
Bleach, 69
Blockages, nasal, 62, 65,
    77, 175, 177–179,
    192–193, 204
Blood clots, 197
Blood pressure, high, 16,
    164, 195, 197
Blood thinners, 195, 196
Blood vessels, 106, 107,
    109, 195
Body temperature, 56, 70
Boek, Wilbert M., 53
Bones
    ethmoid, 134, 175–176,
        178, 204
    maxillary, 204
Botulism, 222
Brain, 12, 134, 164, 182,
    183
Breakfast, in bed, 56
Breath
    bad, 126, 128–130, 217
    shortness of. See Dyspnea.
Breathe-ease XL, 53
Breathe-ease XL Nasal
    Irrigation Solution,
    199

Breathe-ease XL Nasal
    Moisturizing Gel, 68,
    71, 96, 97, 189,
    190–191, 194–195,
    196, 208
Breathe-ease XL Nasal
    Moisturizing Spray,
    171, 189, 190, 196
Breathe Right Nasal Strips,
    193
BreathePure, 47
Breathing, 208
    blocked, 62, 65, 77,
        175, 177–179,
        192–193
    heavy, 158–159
    measured, 12, 50, 77,
        78, 79, 94, 105,
        116–117, 124, 133,
        142, 151–152,
        160–161, 193
    mouth, 138, 218
    nasal, 139, 217–218
Bromelain, 104, 117, 123,
    127, 154, 158, 172,
    218
Bronchioles, 135, 136
Bronchitis, chronic, 146
Bronchoconstriction,
    exercise-induced, 139
Bronchodilators, 140, 150,
    189
Bronchospasms, 141
Bruises, 117
Bruxism, 116
Bulb irrigators, 81–82
Butterbur, 107

Cancer, 164
Carbon dioxide (CO_2),
    149, 185, 186
Carpeting, 48, 69
Cartilage, 204

Cats, 32, 36
Celiac disease, 32–33, 111
Cells, mast, 28, 45, 141
Centers for Disease
    Control (CDC), 10, 68
Cerebrospinal fluid, 134
Cerebrospinal fluid fistula,
    134
Cerebrospinal leak, 134
Chairs, 112
Chantix, 150
Cheese, 112
Chemicals, 184–187
    combustion, 184–185
    dilution of, 188
    household, 69–70
    industrial, 66–67, 196
Chewing gum, 84, 130
Chicken broth, 92
Chicken soup, 76, 92–93,
    200
    recipe, 93
Children, 214–223
Chills, 70, 96, 124
Chlorine, 67, 187
Chlor-Timeton, 44
Chocolate, 112, 115, 195
Chromium, 67, 196
Chronic obstructive
    pulmonary disease
    (COPD), 135, 139,
    146–154
    diagnosing, 149
    medications, 149–150
    symptoms, 147
    whole body approach
    (WBA) to, 149–154
Cilia, 27, 28, 33–34, 51,
    52, 53–54, 57, 67, 70,
    71, 74, 75, 76, 77, 83,
    90, 122, 126, 127, 128,
    135, 136, 185, 188,
    200, 207, 212, 213

measurement of
    movement, 67–68,
    136, 191
Clarinex, 44
Claritin, 44
Cleaning products, 69–70
Clear-ease lozenges, 117,
    127, 158, 161, 172
Closets, 50
Clothes, 47, 70
Coal, 185
Cocaine, 196, 197
Cocoa powder, 195
Coffee, 110
Colds, 62, 70, 71, 88–97,
    206, 214
    complications, 97, 180
    frequency, 97
    prevention, 88
    symptoms, 88, 90
    whole body approach
    (WBA) to, 91–97
Columella, 205
Comedy. See Humor.
Compresses, 122, 200
Computerized tomography
    (CT), 63, 64
Concussions, 178
Congestion, rebound. See
    Rhinitis
    medicamentosa.
Conjunctiva, 110
Conjunctivitis, allergic, 25
Continuous positive air
    pressure (CPAP), 167,
    172, 173, 174
COPD. See Chronic
    obstructive pulmonary
    disease (COPD).
Cortex, 12
Corticosteroids, 150, 210,
    211
Cosmetics, 56

Cough suppressants, 189
Coughs, 55, 56, 61, 139,
    146, 154, 157, 185,
    187, 189, 214, 222
Coumadin, 195
Counterclockwise (Langer),
    79
Cousins, Norman, 7
CPAP. See Continuous
    positive air pressure
    (CPAP).
Cystic fibrosis, 126,
    191–192

Davidson, Terence, 86,
    192
Daxas, 150
Decongestants, 44,
    122–123, 198–200,
    220
    dilution of, 199
Depakote, 108
Depression, 14, 72, 172
Deviated septum. See
    Nasal septum,
    deviated.
Diabetes, 164
Diamox, 107
Diaries
    food, 36, 130, 158
    headache, 105,
    111–112, 123
    sneezing, 34
Didgeridoos. 170
Diesel exhaust, 68
Diets, 142
    elimination, 36–37,
    111, 158
    low-carbohydrate, 130
Diprivan, 170
Discharges, nasal, 21, 36,
    57, 62, 63, 73, 74,
    214, 215

Diseases, autoimmune, 111
Diuretics, 115, 130
Dopamine, 150
Driving, 47
Drugs, 14–16, 33–34
   allergy, 43–45
   interactions, 16
   over-the-counter, 44, 45,
      103, 107, 116, 122,
      127, 141
   prescription, 44–45
   rebound from, 38
   recreational, 190, 195,
      196, 197
   risks, 15–16
Dry mouth. See
   Xerostomia.
Dryness, nasal. See Nose,
   dryness.
Dust, 28–29, 36, 48
   exposure to, 148, 200
Dust mites, 28–29, 48
Dynamic hyperinflation,
   148
Dyspnea, 139–140, 147

Ear tubes. See
   Myringotomy tubes.
Eardrums, 218, 219
Ears, 82, 117, 127, 217,
   218–219
Echinacea, 96
Eczema, 25
Effexor, 108, 177
Elavil, 108
Emphysema, 146
Empty nose syndrome
   (ENS), 83, 207–209
Encasements, 48
Endorphins, 16, 17
Endoscopy, 203, 211
ENS. See Empty nose
   syndrome (ENS).

Enzymes, proteolytic, 117,
   123, 127, 154, 158,
   172
Eosinophils, 26, 65
Epiglottis, 165
EpiPens, 222
Epistaxis. See Nosebleeds.
Estrogen, 115
Ethylamine, 92
Eustachian tube, 82, 217,
   219
Exercises, 105–106, 124,
   148
   cervical neck/shower,
      105, 109–110, 114
   lung strengthening, 142
   smell identification,
      181–182
   smell-recall, 180–181
   throat, 169–170
Exhalation, 136–137,
   138–139, 152
Expiration, 148
Expiratory flow limitation,
   148
Exposures, 23–24, 187
   environmental, 184–189
   whole body approach
      (WBA) to, 187–189
Eye drops, 188
Eyes, 102, 118–119, 188
Eyjafjallajökull, Iceland,
   187

Fasting, 130
FEV1. See Forced
   expiratory volume in
   one second (FEV1).
Fevers, 70
Fight-or-flight response,
   12, 105, 116
Filters
   air, 48

   nose, 47
Flonase, 44, 180, 196
Flossing, 130, 217
Flowback, 81–82, 122
Fluticasone, 140
Flying, 71, 97, 127
Foods, 32–33, 36–37, 57,
   130
Forced expiratory volume
   in one second (FEV1),
   138, 147
Forced vital capacity
   (FVC), 138
Formaldehyde, 69, 200
Fractures, septal, 197
Frenulum, 221
Fruits, citrus, 195
Fungi, 64–65
Furniture, 69

Gargling, 161
Gases, volcanic, 186–187
Gastroesophageal reflux
   disease (GERD), 126,
   131–132, 133, 146,
   158, 164
Ginkgo biloba, 195
Gluten, 32–33, 37, 111
Grandma Josephson's
   Homemade Chicken
   Soup, 93
Grasses, 27, 135
Grossan, Murray,
   144–145, 151–154

Halitosis. See Breathe, bad.
Handwashing, 91
Happy affect, 144
Hawaii, 186
Hay fever. See Rhinitis,
   allergic.
Headaches, 101–124
   amount of pain, 104

circulation (vascular), 109–110
cluster, 110
diagnosing, 119–123
food-related, 111
migraine, 106–108, 115, 120, 177
neck (cervical), 112–113
premenstrual, 115
rhinogenic, 115–116
sinus, 101–103, 119, 121–123
temporomandibular joint disorder (TMJ), 116–117
tension, 105
trigeminal neuralgia, 118
triggers, 108, 111–112
vacuum, 103–104
vision-related, 118–119
whole body approach (WBA) to, 121–123
Healing, 2–3, 7–10, 14–15, 18, 224
Healing places, 153–154
Hearing, 214
Heart disease, 107
Helium, 104
Herbal remedies, 107–108, 123
Hibiscus, 108
Histamines, 18, 23, 28, 41, 44, 56, 112, 141
HIV, 65
Hoarseness, 157–158
Honey, 55, 69, 71, 92, 154, 222
Houser, Steven, 209
Humidification, 121
Humidity, 48–49, 200, 214
Humming, 51, 69, 76, 127, 154, 188, 213

Humor, 7, 11, 16–17, 46–47, 144–145
Hydration. See Water, drinking of.
Hydro-pulse irrigation units, 129, 168–169
Hygiene hypothesis, 24
Hypertension. See Blood pressure, high.
Hyphae, 65
Hyposmia, 176
Hypothalamus, 56

ICAM-1, 70, 71, 90, 95–96
Ig. See Immunoglobulins (Ig).
IgE. See Immunoglobulin E (IgE).
Imitrex, 107
Immune reactions, type 1, 22
Immune system, 11, 23, 24, 72, 87, 144
Immune system cascade, 22
Immunity, 11, 64, 70, 77, 97, 215, 223
Immunoglobulin A (IgA), 23
Immunoglobulin E (IgE), 21–22, 25, 28, 33–34, 52, 111, 112, 126, 141
Immunoglobulin G (IgG), 23
Immunoglobulin M (IgM), 23
Immunoglobulins (Ig), 23, 87
Implants, 108
cochlea, 214
ethmoid, 203, 210

Inderal, 107
Infections, 216
dental, 102
ear. See Otitis media.
sinus. See Sinusitis.
tapeworm, 21
viral, 10, 62, 177, 179, 218
Inflammation, 117, 121, 122, 123, 140, 172
Inflammatory response, 92
Inhalation, 136, 140, 147, 164
steam, 161, 189
Inhalers, 80, 93–94, 189
Injections
desensitization, 22, 28, 34, 35, 43
sclerosing solution, 173
Injuries, head, 178
Inspire, 198, 199
Intal, 141
Interferon, 92
Intracellular adhesion molecule. See ICAM-1.
Irritants, 28

Jackson, Michael, 170
Jacobson, Edmund, 79, 153
Jaws, 116–117, 152
Johnson's Baby Shampoo, 84, 128
Josephson, Jordan, 93, 211–212
Jumping jacks, 69, 127
Jumping rope, 69, 127

Keen, Mark, 81
Kenalog, 110
Ketchup, 112
Ketones, 130
Kilauea, Hawaii, 186

Kinase, 80
Kudrow, Lee, 115

Lactic acid, 114
Lactoferrin, 83
Langer, Ellen, 79
Laryngoscope, 131
Larynx, 127, 157
Laughter, 7, 11, 16, 144
L-cysteine, 92
Lee, John, 82
Lemons, 55, 69, 71, 76, 77, 92, 127, 175, 180
Lenses, transitional, 119
Leukotriene inhibitors, 45, 141
Leukotrienes, 45, 141
Licorice, 112
Lights, 50
Limbic system, 12, 91, 176
Limes, 76, 77, 127, 175
Lipsticks, 56
Lothi, Hawaii, 186
L-theanine, 55, 76, 92, 145
Lump in the throat sensation, 133–134
Lungs, 61, 136, 138–139, 146, 159
Lysozymes, 83

Magnolia flower, 123
Masks
  dust/surgical, 186, 188
  face, 37, 47
  filter, 186, 188
Massages, 124
  cervical neck/shower, 105, 113, 114
Mast cell stabilizers, 45, 141
Mauna Loa, Hawaii, 186

Maxair, 140
Maxalt, 107
Mayonnaise, 112
Medication enhancement, 17–18, 41, 45–47, 54, 146
Medications. See Drugs.
Menthol, 80, 93, 114
Methacholine challenge, 139
Middle meatus, 61
Migraines. See Headaches, migraine.
Migranal, 107
Milk and milk products, 33, 112
Mind, power of, 2–3, 7–10, 14–15, 16, 18, 45–46, 51
Miosis, 110
Mirrors, use of, 50, 78–79, 105, 117, 152, 157, 160
Molds, 29–30, 36, 48, 40–50, 64–65, 200
Monoclonal anti-IgE antibodies, 141
Monosodium glutamate (MSG), 111
Mount Ontake, Japan, 186
Mouth blowing, 169
Mouth guards, 173
Mucinex, 127, 189
Mucus, 27, 51, 61, 71, 76, 117, 125–128, 157–158, 175, 191–192, 219, 220, 222
Mucus membranes, 23, 207
Muscle relaxation, 50, 91, 114, 116–117, 124, 133, 152–154, 160
Muscle tension, 159–160

Muscles, 105, 114, 124
  facial, 91, 159
  frontalis, 152
  jaw, 152, 159
  neck, 159
  smooth, 140, 149
  throat, 133, 155–157, 160–161, 165, 169–170
Mustard, 112
Mycotoxins, 29, 30
Myringotomy tubes, 219, 220
Myringotomy, 219

Naprosyn, 116, 117
Nasal dilator strips, 170, 193
Nasal endoscopes, 73, 211
Nasal gels, 68, 71, 96, 97, 189, 190–191, 194–195
Nasal irrigation, 51, 83, 87, 129, 168–169
  antibiotics and, 85–87, 192
  baby shampoo and, 84, 128
  Proetz, 215
  pulse-wave, 33, 35, 42, 51–55, 65, 70, 80–87, 95–96, 122, 124, 127–128, 143, 168–169, 188, 188, 200, 208, 213, 215
  saline solution and, 52, 53–54, 82–83
  saline solution additions, 83–87, 188
  use of, 54–55, 85
  water type to use, 52–53
  xylitol and, 83–85, 128, 208

Nasal passages, 26–27, 62
    methods of opening, 80,
    94, 170–171, 205
Nasal septum, 61, 204
    deviated, 61, 115, 179,
    192–193, 204–206
    perforated, 196, 197–198
Nasal sprays
    antihistamine, 44, 122
    cortisone, 196
    saline, 71
    steroidal, 44–45, 122
Nasal valve, 170–171
NasalCrom, 45, 141
Nasarel, 196
Nasocort, 196
Nasonex, 44
National Institute for
    Occupational Safety
    and Health (NIOSH),
    186
Neck, 112–114
    cracking, 114
Neosporin, 195
Neo-Synephrine, 198, 199
Neo-Synephrine Extra-
    Strength, 104
Nerves
    facial, 110
    inferior alveolar, 102,
    120
    olfactory, 175–176,
    177–178
    trigeminal, 113, 118,
    119
Nervous system, 77, 110,
    195
Neti pots, 81–82, 122
Neurontin, 108
Neuroplasticity, 9, 78
Niacin, 107, 110, 111
Nickel, 196
NicoDerm, 150

Night guards, 117
Nightlights, 167
Non-allergic rhinitis. See
    Rhinitis, vasomotor/
    non-allergic.
Non-steroidal anti-
    inflammatories
    (NSAIDs), 143, 195
Nose blowing, 66, 77, 96,
    214, 215, 219
Nose drops. See
    Decongestants.
Nose, 26–27, 73, 91,
    115–116, 135, 170,
    193, 208
    crooked, 212
    dryness, 171–172, 175,
    185, 187, 189,
    190–191, 194
    foreign bodies in, 214
    picking, 190, 196
    runny, 26, 27, 57, 110
    stuffy, 38
    tip of, 170–171, 192,
    193, 205
Nosebleeds, 194–197
Nsouli, Talal M., 82

Oils, olive, 112
Olives, 112
Ono, Yoko, 72
Oral hygiene, 130
Oral-antral fistula, 194
Otitis media, 218–220
    acute, 218
    serous, 218
Otrivin, 198, 199
Oxygen, 164
Oz, Mehmet, 81

Pain
    referred from neck,
    112–114, 118, 119

See also Trigeminal
    neuralgia.
Paint thinners/solvents,
    196
Pantosmia, 177
Papain, 104, 117, 123,
    127, 154, 158, 172,
    218
Parosmia, 176–177
Patanase, 44, 130
Peppers, chili, 112
Phenylethylamine, 115
Pheromones, 176
Phosphodiesterase, 150
Phosphodiesterase
    inhibitors, 150
Phosphodiesterase-4
    antagonists, 150
Physical therapy, 105–106
Pickles, 112
Pillar procedure, 173
Placebos, 2, 7–8, 17,
    19–20, 45, 46, 151
Plants, 194
Polio, 114, 177
Pollen calendar, 35–36, 47
Pollens, plant, 25, 26–28,
    34, 35–36, 47, 135
Pollution
    air, 148–149, 184–189
    indoor, 149
    occupational, 148
Polyps, nasal, 44, 60, 65,
    73, 143, 175, 179,
    209, 210, 211–212
Ponaris Nasal Emollient,
    196
Position emission
    tomography (PET)
    scan, 181
Postnasal drip, 125–130,
    157
    symptoms, 126

whole body approach
(WBA) to, 126–128
Posture, 105, 158–159
Prednisone, 199, 210, 211
Pregnancy, 177
Premarin, 191, 208
Prilosec, 132
Probiotics, 64, 66, 70, 87,
97, 223
Prodromata, 106
Progesterone, 115
Proton-pump inhibitors,
132
Proventil, 140
Psychoneuroimmunology,
9, 144, 181
Psychotherapy, 18
Ptosis, 110
Pyridoxine. *See* Vitamin
B$_6$.

Qnasl, 45

Radiation therapy,
129–130
Ragweed, 27
Relaxation, 150, 151–154
progressive, 78–79, 153
Remicade, 150
Respiration, 136
Respiratory system, 40–41,
59
Rhinitis
allergic, 25, 26, 41, 57,
59, 62, 135, 137,
143–144
atrophic, 190–191
vasomotor/non-allergic,
38, 141
Rhinocort, 44
Rhinoplasty, 203, 212
Rhinorrhea. *See* Nose,
runny.

Rhinosinusitis. *See*
Sinusitis.
Rhintitis medicamentosa
(RM), 38, 44,
198–200
Ring of Fire, Pacific
Islands, 187
Ringer's solution, 53
RM. *See* Rhintitis
medicamentosa (RM).
Rutin, 195

Saccharin, 67–68, 191
Saddle nose deformity,
197, 198
Saline solutions, 52,
53–54, 82–83
Saliva, 130
Salivary glands, 129
Salt, 115
Samter's triad, 143
Sansert, 107
Scuba diving, 104, 127
Sensodyne ProNamel, 55,
77
Septoplasty, 203, 204–206
Serevent Discus, 140
Serous fluid, 219
Shoes, 47
Shoulders, 152–153
Shower curtains, 49
Showers, 107, 121
Sialidnitis, 129
Sick building syndrome,
30, 200
Signals, 78, 79, 95, 152,
153
Silica, 148
Silicosis, 148
Simple Saline, 171, 189
Singing, 157, 158,169,
221
Singulair, 45, 141

Sinuplasty, 209
balloon, 203, 210
Sinus Relief Now
(Josephson), 211–212
Sinuses, 60–61, 82, 136,
209
ethmoid, 60, 73, 102,
120
frontal, 60–61, 73, 102,
210
maxillary, 60, 61, 73,
102, 120, 194, 210
methods of opening,
104
sphenoid, 61, 102–103,
120
Sinusitis, 2, 11, 19, 33–34,
41, 59–87, 135, 137,
143–144, 146, 180,
196, 217
acute, 62–63, 215
children's, 215–216
chronic, 34, 41, 57,
63–64, 75, 81, 84–85,
137, 143–144, 179,
209, 215
diagnosing, 72–73
fungal, 30, 64–66
pan, 209
prevention, 59, 66–73
symptoms, 62, 63, 73,
75, 89, 102–103,
120–121
treatment, 74–87
whole body approach
(WBA) to, 66–73,
75–87, 121–123
Skiing, 116
Skin, 151, 152, 153, 195
Sleep, 11, 14, 72, 77, 80,
93–94, 124, 130, 164,
165, 167
depression and, 172

Sleep apnea, 164, 222
children and, 222–223
depression and, 172
surgical corrections for,
172–173
testing for, 167
treatments, 167,
172–173
SLIT. *See* Sublingual
immunization therapy
(SLIT).
Smell, 175–176, 181
loss of, 96, 176,
177–179
whole body approach
(WBA) to, 180–183
Smiling, 11, 16, 72, 91,
97, 144, 224
Smog, 68–69, 185–186
Smoking, 135, 146, 148,
149
Smoking cessation,
150–154
medications, 150
whole body approach
(WBA) to, 150–154
Sneezing, 56, 96
Snoring, 163–174
causes, 166
children and, 166, 214,
218
whole body approach
(WBA) to, 168–174
Soft palate, 163, 165, 173,
218
Somnoplasty, 173
Songs, 221
Soundboards, 127
Soy sauce, 112
Speech, 161–162
delayed, 221
Spiriva, 149–150
Spirometry, 138–139, 149

Sprays, saline, 171
Sprinklers, 49
Squinting, 118
Stachybotrys chartarum, 30
Stem cells, 180–181
Stomach acid, 126, 132,
146, 158, 164
Stress and stress reduction,
3, 11–13, 17–18, 50,
72, 77–80, 94–95,
105, 116, 124, 133,
144, 150–154
*Stressed? Anxiety? Your Cure
Is in the Mirror*
(Grossan), 144–145,
151–154
Sublingual immunization
therapy (SLIT), 43
Submucous resection, 203,
207
Sudafed, 44, 122–123
Sulfites, 112
Sulfur dioxide (SO$_2$), 185,
186
Sulfuric acid, 148–149, 185
Sunglasses, 119
Surfactin, 84, 128
Surgeries, 203–213
explanation of, 42
image-guided, 203,
209–210
rewards and, 42
whole body approach
(WBA) to, 213
Swallowing, 133, 173
Sweeteners, artificial, 112
Swimming, 220
Symbicort, 140

T cells, gamma-delta, 92
Taste, 177, 222
Teas, 56, 70, 71, 92, 97,
200, 213

green and black, 56, 76,
92, 145, 154, 188, 195
hibiscus, 108–109
with lemon and honey,
55, 69, 71, 127
oolong, 195
peppermint, 71
Teeth, 55, 73, 77, 116,
120, 130, 194
Temporomandibular joint
disorder (TMJ),
116–117
Tenderness, 73
Thalamus, 12
Theolair, 150
Throat clearing, 139, 157
Throat irrigation, 129,
168, 217
Throat tickles, 131–132,
139, 157
Tichenor, Wellington, 53,
65
Tiger's Balm, 114
TMJ. *See* Temporoman-
dibular joint disorder
(TMJ).
Tobradex, 86
Tongue, 129, 165, 169, 221
Tongue-suspension
procedure, 173
Tonsillectomy, 216
Tonsillitis, 216
Tonsilloliths, 168, 217
Tonsils, 163, 165, 168, 216
enlarged, 216–217, 223
lingual, 165
Toothpaste, 55, 77
Treatments
drug-free, 9–10, 11
early, 2, 10
patient participation in,
3, 7–10, 19, 45–47,
224

Trees, 27
Trigeminal neuralgia, 118
Trumpets, 170
Tumor necrosis factor
    (TNF) antagonists,
    150
Turbinate reduction, 203,
    206–207
Turbinates, 61, 67–68,
    115, 204–205,
    206–209
    inferior, 61, 192, 204
    middle, 61
Turbinectomy, 203, 207

Unified airway theory, 40,
    89, 136
Urticaria, 141
Uvula, 163, 165, 168
Uvulopalatopharyngoplasty,
    173

Vacations, 48
Vacuuming, 48
Vagus nerve reflexes, 141
Vaporizers, 171, 195
Vasodilators, 110, 111
Ventilation, 49
Vibrations, 165–166, 188
Vinegar, 112
Viruses, 88, 89–90, 92

Visualization, 11, 13,
    17–18, 41–42, 45,
    54–55, 78, 79, 94–95,
    152, 153–154
Vitamin B$_3$. See Niacin.
Vitamin B$_6$, 180
Vitamin C, 195
Vitamins, multi- , 111
Vocal cords, 131,
    139,155–157, 161
Vocal technique, 156
Voice, 155–162
    disorders, 139, 157–160
    symptoms, 156
    whole body approach
    (WBA) to, 160–162
Voice lessons, 161–162
Voice-to-text dictation,
    161–162
Volatile organic
    compounds, 69
Volcanoes, 186–187

Walking, 106
Water, drinking of, 11,
    76–77, 127, 130, 158,
    188, 189
Water retention, 115
WBA. See Whole body
    approach (WBA).
Weeds, 27
Weight, 163, 167

Wheat, 32, 111
Wheezing, 137
Whole body approach
    (WBA), 7–20, 41,
    66–73, 75–87, 91–97,
    121–123, 126–128,
    140–146, 149–154,
    160–162, 168–174,
    180–183, 187–189,
    213, 224
Wildfires, 184–185, 186
Window treatments, 48
Wine, red, 111
World Health
    Organization, 10

Xerostomia, 129
Xolair, 141
Xylitol, 83–85, 196
Xyzal, 44

Yeasts, 64–65
Yogurt, 64, 66, 70, 87, 97,
    223

Zestril, 107
Zinc, 96, 177
Zomig, 107
Zyban, 150
Zyflo, 141
Zyrtec, 44

ABOUT THE AUTHOR

Murray Grossan, M.D., is a board-certified otolaryngologist and head and neck surgeon at Cedars-Sinai in Los Angeles. Well known for his many innovations in sinus and allergy therapy, Dr. Grossan is the founder of Hydro Med Inc. that markets his Hydro Pulse nasal and sinus irrigator, which *Time* magazine called the "Invention of the Year" in 2000. Dr. Grossan has talked about his whole body approach and drug-free methods for resolving allergy and sinus conditions on radio and television, and in peer-review medical journals and such popular books as *The Sinus Cure* (2001) and *Free Yourself from Sinus and Allergy Problems Permanently* (2009). He contributes regularly to the publications *Bottom Line Health* and *Bottom Line Personal,* and has a blog at www.grossaninstitute.com. Dr. Grossan is on the recommended referral list of the Divers Alert Network and the American Tinnitus Association.